CYPRUS AND INTERNATIONAL PEACEMAKING

FARID MIRBAGHERI

Cyprus and International Peacemaking

Routledge
Taylor & Francis Group
New York London

First published in 1998 by

Routledge
711 Third Avenue
New York, NY 10017

Routledge
2 Park Square, Milton Park
Abingdon, Oxon, OX14 4RN

Cataloging in Publication data available from the Library of Congress

ISBN 0-415-91975-4

PREFACE AND ACKNOWLEDGEMENTS

Cyprus is the third largest Mediterranean island. It is situated south of Turkey, west of Syria, north of Egypt and east of Greece. It covers 9,251 square kilometres and has a population of around 800,000. Its history spans nearly 8,000 years – a turbulent story of conquest for some and defeat for others. The two main communities are of Greek and Turkish origin, 80 per cent and 18 per cent respectively. The remaining 2 per cent is composed of Maronites, Armenians and others. Since 1945, Cyprus has been deeply affected by the animosity between the two mother countries, Greece and Turkey. The Cyprus problem has been on the international political agenda for more then three decades. Despite numerous international efforts to find a peaceful resolution the conflict is still very much alive in the 1990s.

There are many facets to the problem, but two are especially notable. The first is internal: the inability of the Greek and Turkish communities in Cyprus to agree on a solution that safeguards the interests of both. The second aspect is international: the involvement of Greece, Turkey and Britain (guarantor powers of the 1960 Cyprus independence constitution) in the dispute. Because of this, and because of old rivalries between Greece and Turkey and the consequent risk both pose to international peace and security, Cyprus has received and continues to receive international attention seemingly out of proportion to its size and population.

This book deals with international peacemaking efforts to resolve the Cyprus problem between 1964 and 1986 and investigates why they failed. It covers the attempts of the United Nations and various states, including the United States and Britain. It focuses particularly on the question of intercommunal mistrust as an important contributing factor, which some believe lies at the root of the problem, and which showed itself in the first three years of the Republic of Cyprus, 1960-3. As one observer noted, 'In the disputes over the application of the Zurich and London agreements, a heavy burden of mutual suspicion and fear had been created.'[1]

The book consists of six chapters. The first deals with the experience of the UN in peacemaking generally, with some observations on its efforts in Cyprus in particular. Since the UN has been the main agency entrusted with bringing about a peaceful solution and an agreed settlement to the Cyprus problem, the first chapter outlines the role and the capacity of the world organisation as the global peacemaking body. Chapter 2 gives a general background to the problem up to December 1963, when it began to attract more acute international attention and the UN was asked to mediate in the dispute. Why the institutions of government in Cyprus broke down in 1963 are described in this chapter. The first phase of the UN's involvement in the immediate aftermath of the 1963 crisis is outlined in Chapter 3. This chapter offers an analysis of the Galo Plaza Report on Cyprus and its reception by the two communities. Chapter 4 covers international peacemaking efforts in Cyprus from 1964 to 1974. Here the core event is the crisis of November 1967, with the intercommunal talks that followed and continued intermittently till 1974. The military coup of 1967 in Greece, and its impact on Cyprus and international peacemaking efforts up to 1974, are outlined. Chapter 5 deals with the most crucial events of the modern period: the Greek-staged coup in the island in 1974 and the subsequent invasion by Turkey. These events changed the balance of forces in Cyprus, and as a result international peacemaking efforts started on a new basis. The efforts of outside powers, namely the American-British-Canadian initiative in the late 1970s, and the two intercommunal High-Level Agreements of 1977 and 1979, are outlined. The sixth and last chapter covers the seven years 1980-6. Unquestionably this period witnessed the most active UN peacemaking efforts in Cyprus. Perhaps this was partly due to the arrival in 1982 of a new UN Secretary-General, Javier Pérez de Cuéllar, who had first-hand knowledge of the Cyprus problem, having been the special representative of the UN Secretary-General in Cyprus in the 1970s. Also during this period there were signs that the United States government fully and actively supported the UN's endeavours to bring about a peaceful solution. In the conclusion an effort is made to analyse the whole international peacemaking effort in Cyprus between 1964 and 1986, relating it to the difficulties posed by the intercommunal mistrust on the island and to the role of interested outsiders. The conclusion also proposes a way forward for peacemaking in Cyprus, by indicating how its weaknesses could be overcome and how the opportunities for a peaceful solution could be enhanced.

Notes

1. Robert Stephens, *Cyprus A place of Arms*, London: Pall Mall Press, 1966, p.182.

Acknowledgements

I am indebted to a number of people for their help in completing this book. First, I owe thanks to my parents for supporting me wholeheartedly throughout the years I have been studying. Without their generous and uninterrupted support, financial and otherwise, this work would have been impossible. I shall never be able to thank them enough. Professor Alan James, research professor and former head of the International Relations department at Keele University, has played a crucial and indispensable role in the completion of this study. As my principal supervisor, his comments have been pivotal; he also facilitated my visits to various United Nations centres and I shall be indebted to him all my life. I would like to thank deeply Dan Keohane, senior lecturer in the International Relations department, Keele University, who as my acting supervisor devoted much time and effort to assisting me, and this study has benefited from his comments and guidelines. I also thank Christopher Brewin, senior lecturer in the same department, for helping with comments on the earlier part of this work.

A number of people granted me the opportunity to interview them and helped me with my inquiries. Some of them do not wish to be identified but I wish to express my thanks and appreciation to all of them, and to others with whom I corresponded. I must mention by name Mr Glafkos Clerides, President of Cyprus; Mr Ozker Ozgur, former leader of the Turkish Republican Party; Mr Sotiris Georgalis of the Cyprus High Commission, London; Mr Alpay Gench, formerly of the Office of the 'Turkish Republic of Northern Cyprus'; Mr Martin Wattam, formerly of the Information Centre in London; the late Brigadier Michael Harbottle; Mr Charles Goulkin, former Spokesman of UNFICYP; Dr Peter Loizos, London School of Economics; Professor Glen Camp, Bryant College, Rhode Island; and Dr Carl Grundy-Warr, formerly of Durham University.

I would also like to thank all those with whom I communicated about this work.

I owe thanks to many institutions, including Keele University Library; the British Library in London; the Public Records Office at Kew; the Public and Information Office, Nicosia; the Cyprus Research Centre, Nicosia; the United Nations Information Centre, London; the United Nations Library, Geneva; the Archives Unit, United Nations, New York; the Cyprus High Commission, London; and the Royal Institute of International Affairs, Chatham House, London.

Last, but not least, I express my deepest gratitude and highest regard to my wife, Maria. I thank her for offering impartial advice on the sources I have used and facilitating some of the interviews, also for the frequent lonely hours that she endured while I was engaged on this work. But most of all I thank her for the love and vital support that kept me persevering even at the most difficult times.

Understandably, some of those who I interviewed or who otherwise assisted me may disagree with some or all of the contents, but this in no way lessens my gratitude to them. The book gives my own interpretation of events and I alone am responsible for any errors, factual or otherwise.

London, September 1997 F. M.

CONTENTS

MAPS

CHRONOLOGY OF CYPRUS SINCE INDEPENDENCE

1960	
16 August	Independence
1963	
30 November	Archbishop Makarios's Thirteen Proposals for Constitutional amendments
20 December	Beginning of intercommunal violence
1964	
4 March	UN Security Council Resolution 186
26 March	Submission of the Plaza Report
27 March	Beginning of UNFICYP operation in Cyprus
1967	
21 April	Military regime seizes power in Greece
15 November	The crisis of November 1967
1968	
24 June-28 August	First phase of the 1968-74 Intercommunal Talks
1969	
29 August 1968-3 January	Second phase of the 1968-74 Intercommunal Talks
1969-1970	Third phase of the 1968-74 Intercommunal Talks
1970	
21 September-July 1974	Fourth phase of the 1968-74 Intercommunal Talks
1974	
15 July	Greek-staged coup in Cyprus
20 July	Turkish invasion (first phase)
22 July	Collapse of military regime in Greece and of puppet regime in Cyprus
25-30 July	First round of Geneva Talks
8-14 August	Second round of Geneva Talks
14 August	Turkish invasion (second phase)
1975	
13 February	Unilateral declaration of Turkish Federated State of Kibris (TFSK) by Turkish Cypriots

28 April-3 May	First round of Vienna Talks (first series)
5-7 June	Second round of Vienna Talks (first series)
31 July-2 August	Third round of Vienna Talks (first series)
8-10 September	Fourth round of Vienna Talks (first series)
1976	
17-21 February	Fifth round of Vienna Talks (first series)
1977	
12 February	High-Level Agreement between Makarios and Denktash
31 March-7 April	Second series of Vienna Talks
1977	
3 August	Death of Archbishop Makarios
1978	
November	The American-British-Canadian Initiative
1979	
19 May	High-Level Agreement between Kyprianou and Denktash
Winter of 1980-1	UN Secretary-General's 'Interim Agreement Proposal'
1981	
22 October	The UN's 'Gobbi Initiative'
1983	
August	UN Secretary-General's Initiative
15 November	Unilateral Declaration of Independence of 'Turkish Republic of Northern Cyprus' (TRNC)
1984	
7 August	UN Secretary-General's Vienna 'Working Points'
1985	
10 September-20 January	'Proximity Talks'
1986	
29 March	UN Secretary-General's 'Draft Framework Agreement'

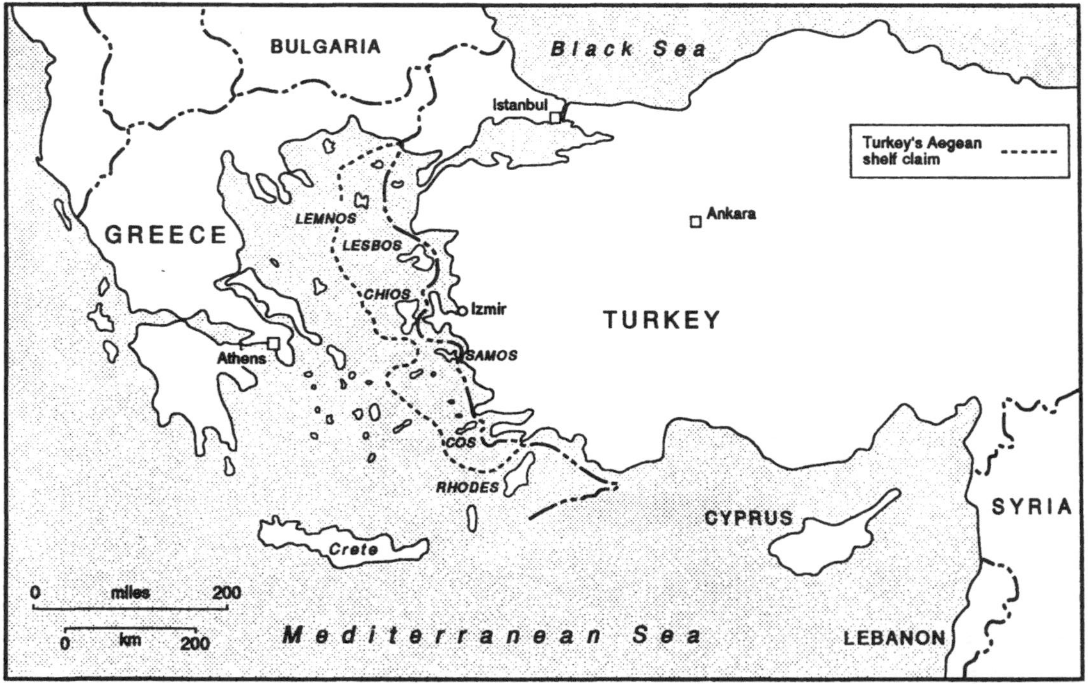

The Eastern Mediterranean

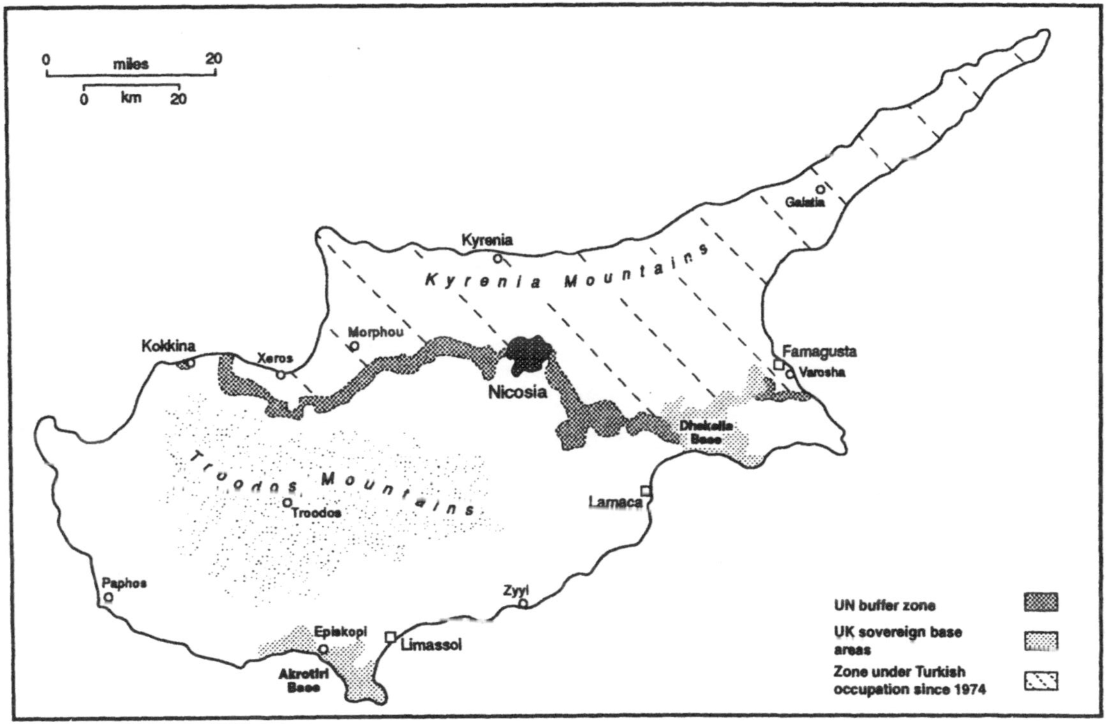

Cyprus since 1974

1

MEDIATION AND THE UNITED NATIONS

'The parties to any dispute, the continuance of which is likely to endanger the maintenance of international peace and security, shall, first of all, seek a solution by negotiation, enquiry, mediation, conciliation, arbitration, judicial settlement, resort to regional agencies, or arrangements, or other peaceful means of their own choice.'[1]

What is mediation?

Mediation is an art and not a science. As a branch of diplomacy used to settle or resolve disputes among conflicting parties it is important in its own right. Although certain elements are necessary when intermediary assistance is to be applied, there is no set of rules or laws which allows any certainty about the outcome. Compared with other forms of conflict resolution, such as arbitration or adjudication, mediation is less formal and more flexible. It seeks to accommodate conflicting interests by persuasion and the exchange of concessions rather than by determination of the rights and obligations involved. There are no procedural requirements as such, and the consent of the parties is essential throughout. And it is flexible because the negotiations can be tailored to suit each occasion as the circumstances may demand.

Mediation can be either passive or active. Passive mediation seeks to bring the disputants together in the presence of a third party. In the active mode a mediator participates at some stage to effect a settlement by undertaking some responsibilities. UN mediation in Cyprus since 1965 in the role of the special representative of the Secretary-General exemplifies the passive category of mediation.[2] The role played by Ellsworth Bunker in the West Irian controversy in 1962 represents the active category.[3]

Certain features associated with the mediatory process distinguish it from other kinds of conflict resolution. First, since all mediation involves negotiations among the conflicting parties themselves, as well as between them and the intermediary, the granting of concessions from both sides is an essential requirement. Of course this may place certain limitations on the mediator, and here too informality and flexibility as needed. Another important feature of the process is that it does not carry a sense of finality in the determination of the rights and obligations of the parties. This encourages the disputants to seek intermediary assistance, because they do not see themselves committed to any particular solution by virtue of having asked for it.

Also central to the diplomatic forum of mediation is the endeavour to develop perceptions of common interest. As put by one writer:

> In international mediation, the peace-maker's function is not to expound to those involved an indivisible, immutable truth, but to help them create a new truth about their relationships by finding firm ground for agreements that will benefit both parties and bring their vital interests into closer harmony.[4]

The importance attributed by parties to what they initially asserted to be vital does at times suggest the improbability of accommodating their conflicting claims. The following aspect of the India-Pakistan question illustrates this point:

> The Minister for Foreign Affairs [of Pakistan] dwelt at length on economic and strategic considerations. He argued that India, if it has control of Jammu and Kashmir, would be in a position to divert all five rivers of the Punjab...Jhelum, under Indian control and thus could reduce to a desert one-third of the irrigated areas of the west Punjab.[5]

The Indian government replied:

> the strategic interests of a country like India, with its big land mass in the Indian Ocean, are at least as vital in the world as the strategic interest of its neighbour.[6]

These incompatible claims were later reconciled through the submission of alternative proposals by a mediator in the India-Pakistan dispute, Sir Owen Dixon, who attempted to narrow the areas of interest each held to be of 'strategic importance'.[7]

Maintaining the confidentiality of negotiations is another important aspect of intermediary assistance, as premature disclosure of the position of the disputants may lead to domestic pressure in their home countries. This means that governments find it very difficult to retreat from positions which have been made public.

In such cases concessions, which are often essential to any successful mediation, are not forthcoming. The conflicting parties may even succumb to the temptation of making capital at home at the risk of failure in the negotiations by taking public positions and stubbornly adhering to them. However, when confidentiality is observed, parties feel free to approach the mediator with their genuine views of the problems in dispute. This aspect has a significant bearing on the case of Cyprus, as will be explained in the following chapters.

Observing, clarifying and elaborating are all routine procedures of the intermediary process. This can provide the background to concessions and rationalise them by justifying the reasons for them. One writer has noted:

> The mere fact of a mediator's entrance into a dispute provides the parties with a means for rationalising retreats from previously held positions, particularly if the mediator can be made to appear to take part of the responsibility for any settlement.[8]

Factors affecting the outcome of mediation

Once parties in dispute accept third-party assistance, certain factors come into play to shape the outcome. Some of these factors relate to the conflict itself and some to the performance of the mediator. The most important of them are identified below.

Advantages gained on the battlefield are an important bargaining-counter at the negotiating table. The party that has the upper hand militarily may only be willing to negotiate if it anticipates political gains from this advantage. By the same token the weaker side may be unyielding to pressure for talks from outside until the balance in the military arena has been restored. In such cases, obtaining the consent of the disputants for third party assistance may prove a difficult and lengthy task.

Some conflicts are potentially more threatening to international peace and security than others. The degree of involvement by world or regional superpowers is an index of the dangers inherent in such conflicts, and is a factor which cannot be ignored by the third party. A mediator also has to take into account the gravity of the situation and the nature of the conflict. All these considerations are important when devising the appropriate procedure for negotiations.

'Concretisation of issues' is also important: a clear understanding of the various claims of the mediator and the parties themselves is needed to establish common ground. Issues must be clearly defined and separated from one another, and when necessary redefined by the mediator to help bring about new perceptions of the parties' common interest.[9] Sometimes this change of perception is essential to the whole process of mediation, as the disputants tend to view their conflict in zero-sum terms.[10]

Before any attempt at mediation is made, a cease-fire must be established, since a continuation of hostilities is usually seen as incompatible with negotiations. For example, in the Indonesian situation the success of the Committee of Good Offices in bringing about a settlement was said to depend on the prior establishment of a truce.

> It seems obvious that an effective truce is a prerequisite to fruitful negotiations and that therefore the effectiveness of our Committee of Good Offices will be substantially prejudiced by the failure of the parties to reach an agreement regarding the cessation of hostilities.[11]

When in 1948 the UN Security Council appointed a commission to find out the facts of the Kashmir dispute and lend its good offices to India and Pakistan, it called on the governments of both countries 'to take immediately all measures within their power...to refrain from making any statement and from doing or causing to be done or permitting any acts which might aggravate the situation'.[12]

Although sought for its own sake, a cease-fire naturally does not imply a resolution of the conflict, but it may pave the way for a comprehensive arrangement which will eventually lead to one. As a means of conflict resolution a cease-fire does not in itself stand much of a chance and can be very fragile. Ideally, there will be a close link between cease-fire proposals and an agreement to negotiate on the underlying differences. For instance, the cease-fire proposals in the India-Pakistan case in 1965 were viewed by Pakistan as deficient because procedures for settlement of the dispute were not agreed at the same time.[13]

Any mediator must maintain the confidence of the parties in order to remain a viable channel of communication for the disputants to exchange views. The parties to a conflict are more likely to approach a prospective mediator, confident that their bargaining positions during negotiation will not be turned against them.

The proper conduct of intermediary procedures requires the participation of all parties to a dispute. As the long-term effectiveness of a settlement may largely depend on the degree to which it commands their cooperation, participation by all the interested parties becomes imperative for success. The absence of an interested party may thus weaken the authority of the decisions reached. A classic example is the failure of early mediation attempts in Cyprus. In March 1957 Paul H. Spaak, then Secretary-General of the North Atlantic Treaty Organisation (NATO), offered to mediate between Britain, Greece and Turkey – all members of NATO and directly concerned with the fate of Cyprus. However this offer was rejected by Greece on the ground that no settlement could come about without a representative of the Cypriot people participating. Turkey, on the other hand, was adamantly opposed to any negotiation that included Archbishop Makarios, the Greek Cypriot leader, and threatened to boycott it.[14]

'Negotiability' is a term which refers to various aspects of bargaining.

Usually, when a party claims that an issue is not negotiable, it means that achievement of its objective is more important than an agreed settlement of that particular issue with the other disputants.[15] The mediator's task in such cases is to persuade the party to change its perception that the problems are not subject to discussion and compromise.[16] 'Non-negotiability' could then mean that alternative approaches to the achievement of the goals, in a manner satisfactory to both parties, have not been explored. Obviously, there could be no room for any compromise if one or more of the parties assert that none of the issues in question are negotiable.[17] In such cases the mediator might help the disputants reorient their claims by seeking possible inputs and reinforcements from sources outside the immediate area of conflict.[18] Pressure applied by powers whose views the disputants must heed is an extremely useful tool in bringing them to the negotiating table.[19] However, if all the intermediary's efforts fail to affect the uncompromising position of the parties, an indefinite stalemate may result, leading to claims that the status quo be legitimised. This has been an issue of concern in the case of Cyprus, as is explained later.

The personality and conduct of the proposed mediator may also affect the willingness of the conflicting parties to resort to the process and allow him sufficient room to manoeuvre for a negotiated settlement. The extent of a mediator's personal capability and authority are of such character, and skill, charisma and impartiality are influential factors in the parties' evaluation of him or her. In practice, however, the mediator's ability to command external support for his efforts may play an even more important role.

As for the success of intermediary assistance, several factors have to be taken into account. One is the official competence of the decision-mechanism – whether or not a third party's decisions or recommendations are likely to be heeded by the disputants and, more broadly, by the outside world. Another factor is the appropriateness of the procedures to the particular requirements of the case in point. The degree and nature of formal authority that the intermediary brings to bear can also influence the outcome. Finally, the deference accorded to intermediary authority can affect the degree of success attainable by such peacemaking procedures.

The United Nations as a mediator in international disputes

Before parties to a dispute decide to resort to the United Nations for third-party assistance, they are likely to consider all the possible ramifications. One of the most obvious consequences of such action is the internationalisation of the problem. This may affect the interest of one or the other of disputants adversely, since UN involvement may lend additional legitimacy to a claim and thus alter the balance of the parties' relative bargaining power. There are other grounds too on which internationalisation of a problem may be strongly resisted, even by parties not directly involved. For instance in the Cyprus case, the US government was strongly opposed before independence to any recourse to the UN contrary to the wishes of the Greek government: internationalising the case would have magnified the rift between Greece and Turkey, both members of NATO, and this would have embarrassed Washington.

The question of whether the UN should become involved is also influenced by expectations concerning the outcome. These may stem from the structure and composition of the UN organs at the time, and the standards by which the claims of the parties will be evaluated. The intrusion of the UN may thus be viewed as unhelpful in devising a prompt, just and effective settlement.

Recourse to the UN and the appointment of a mediator in themselves usually reflect advance agreements by the parties to that effect. A basis for such agreements is catered for in the UN, for example through the Security Council, its principal organ for dealing with conflict situations. Because of its non-judicial status, when considering a question under Chapter VI of the Charter the Security Council can offer parties a flexible framework which may help them to reach a compromise. Even when the parties wish to avoid Security Council involvement, they can still benefit fully from the UN's informal good offices. An example of this may be seen in the way it handled the expulsion of persons of Asian origin from Uganda, where the good offices of the Secretary-General and of other interested member states within the region made a useful contribution.[20] As for the appropriate procedures for settling a conflict, parties involved are free to choose any procedure that appeals to them. On occasion, the mediator's task is to persuade the parties to settle their differences through peaceful means other than mediation, for instance judicial methods, as in the case of the Jarring Report in the India-Pakistan question.[21]

There are certain accepted norms in the practice of peacemaking and mediation by the UN. First and foremost, the mediator should not act in a manner contrary to its purposes and principles as stated in Article 1 of the UN Charter. If this proves an impossible task, the mediator may have to withdraw and return his mandate to the parent organ.

Although the UN cannot prescribe the terms and conditions of a settlement, the participation of its appointed mediator in the negotiations makes it most likely that any settlement reached will enjoy the support of the international community. Hence it is incumbent on the mediator to ensure that the agreed settlement is not contrary to the fundamental principles of justice and international law. It was over this principle that Javier Pérez de Cuéllar, when acting as the then Secretary-General's special representative in Cyprus stated:

> It [any settlement] must be consistent with the provisions of the United Nations Charter, of which the following in particular seems relevant: the purposes, principles and obligations relating to the maintenance of international peace and security, the peaceful settlement of disputes, respect for the principle of equal rights and self-determination of peoples, respect for human rights and fundamental freedoms, recognition of sovereign equality of member states, abstention from the threat or use of force against the territorial integrity or political independence of any state, and respect for treaty obligations not in conflict with those of the member states under the Charter.[22]

When a dispute is put before the UN at a highly inflammable stage, the priority is to prevent an outbreak or recurrence of fighting, or to establish a cease-fire. Direct intrusion into issues in dispute is avoided so that the parties feel secure enough to submit to the UN's will. For instance, in the conflict between India and Pakistan in 1965 the UN Secretary-General offered his good offices to the disputants to establish an immediate cease-fire.[23] However, when reporting to the Security Council he pointed out that this involved no judgement on his part on the merits of the dispute:

> As Secretary-General, my primary concern at this stage has been necessarily with the current breaches of the cease-fire agreement and the CFL. There is, of course, a long and extensive background to the Kashmir problem of which the cease-fire agreement is but one aspect.[...] Thus, reference to the political factors in the broad Kashmir issue, past and present, and political assessments or judgements are avoided here. Though fully aware of the political factors, and their implications, I could not presume to act as political arbiter.[24]

The question of coordination between various organs of the United Nations assumes considerable importance once mediation is formally under way. This problem is reflected in a statement made by the Palestine Commission in the late 1940s:

> The sole motivation of the commission is to obtain from the Security Council that effective assistance without which, it is firmly convinced, it cannot discharge the great responsiblities entrusted to it by the General Assembly.[25]

In this case, although the Palestine Commission was the result of a General Assembly Resolution (181 [II]), it lacked the necessary assistance from the Security Council, and the problem of coordination remained even after the Palestine Commission was replaced by a mediator.

The degree of parties' confidence in the UN's procedures also plays an important role in the process of mediation. If the disputing parties can be assured that the outcome is likely to be just as well as effective, and to respond to their common interests, they are more likely to cooperate fully with its appointed mediator – whatever the balance of advantage at the moment of cease-fire.

Before it can begin negotiations, the UN urges the conflicting parties to agree to a cease-fire. The assistance that it can provide in this case may take the form of peacekeeping. UN peacekeeping forces are, at any time, stationed in a number of parts of the world where a settlement between the disputing parties is lacking but with their consent, in order to help maintain peace and security. However, there are suggestions that this sort of UN presence tends to freeze the attitudes of the parties and hence delay a settlement. Here the classic case is Cyprus where, since 1964, UNFICYP (United Nations Forces in Cyprus) has tried to prevent violence between the two communities and maintain order. Yet the parties have not compromised throughout the years of the UNFICYP presence. Whether or not this argument is true in every case, the fact remains that for a negotiated settlement to be reached hostilities must come to an end and the UN, as the body entrusted by member states and the international community, must seek to achieve this. However, to avoid the freezing of attitudes by the parties, it may be best to establish a close link between peacekeeping and peacemaking proposals.

There are occasions when a dispute falls exclusively within a state's reserved domain which Article 2(7) of the UN Charter recognises as embracing 'matters which are essentially within the domestic jurisdiction of any state'. In these cases the UN has no authority to intervene (except in circumstances covered under chapter VII), nor are states under any obligation to submit them for settlement to the UN. However, certain kinds of internal conflict are potentially threatening to international peace and security and must be outside the reserved domain. It has now been accepted by most member states that racial discrimination, mass killings and expulsions, and the like are no longer matters exclusively within the domestic jurisdiction of the states that practise them.[26] It is important to note that historically the gap between the notions of 'interest' and 'principles' has narrowed. This was manifested in the United States military operation in 1992 to provide aid in Somalia. Since the way interest and principles interrelate is subject to historical change, the UN, in offering intermediary assistance in a dispute, cannot but be affected by such changes.

When the UN does offer such assistance, it may have to establish contacts with non-sovereign entities, especially in controversies where the question of self-determination affecting territorial sovereignty is at the core of the problem. Sometimes, however, it is difficult to ensure the participation of such parties. In the East Pakistan crisis of 1971 the Secretary-General failed to get the representatives of East Pakistan, as it then was, to participate in the negotiations.[27] Furthermore, in mediating between disputing parities, the UN tries to avoid prejudicing the world community where the sovereignty of the parties is concerned. Recognition of this principle was explicit in the Indonesian question. When putting the question of whether or not to invite the representative of Indonesia to the vote in the Security Council in 1947, the President of the Security Council stated that he did so 'without any definition or determination of the sovereignty of the republic of Indonesia'. He went on to observe that 'every member retains complete liberty either to recognise or not to recognise the sovereignty or independence of the Indonesian Republic'.[28]

In the resolution of disputes through mediation, the mandates issued by the UN provide the framework within which settlements are to be sought. These are sometimes very specific in indicating the terms of a settlement, which may close doors to alternative approaches. There are examples that show both the success and the failure of specific mandates. Resolution S/1234 of 28 January 1949 on the Indonesian situation is an instance of success; Resolution S/726 of 21 April 1948, on the India-Pakistan situation failed. Thus a specific mandate, while clarifying the issues in dispute and clearly introducing the criteria for this resolution, may obstruct the later introduction of alternative bases necessary for further progress.

When seeking such alternative bases for securing a settlement, it may become necessary for the mediator to broaden his terms of reference, to which the parties will also need to agree. The assumption here is that if the original premises for working out a settlement are unworkable, a new approach has to be adopted.[29] However this could present a problem as one or the other of the parties may see it as damaging to their interests. The following statement by Galo Plaza, the UN mediator in Cyprus in the 1964-5 period, elucidates this point:

> I have considered very carefully the meaning to be attached to my terms of reference. Clearly my first duty was...to undertake consultations with each of the parties concerned in order to explore the possibility of their reaching agreement among themselves. I have done that and it has led me to believe that without a change in present circumstances, no such possibility exists. It has accordingly been suggested to me, by some of the parties concerned, that my next responsibility is to bring forward in this report my own proposals for those conditions of settlement which, in my opinion, would allow the parties to go as close as circumstances permit to their legitimate

objectives. But another of the parties has contended that any such proposals, especially since they would in a sense bear the stamp and accordingly the moral force of the United Nations, would tend to place me in the position of an arbitrator rather than a mediator and therefore to carry me beyond the limits of my terms of reference.[...] I do not necessarily accept that contention.[30]

Recourse to UN assistance usually takes place well after the possibilities for reaching a settlement by direct negotiation between the parties have been fully exhausted, as in the cases of Kashmir, Cyprus and the Middle East. In general, however, the presence of the UN in a dispute is likely to minimise tension. As the UN Secretary-General noted in his 1973 annual report, 'Conflict situations, or potential conflict situations, where the United Nations has been involved have tended to be far less violent and destructive than those where it has not been involved, even when the organisation has been unable to effect a settlement of the basic problems concerned.'[31]

Mediation is difficult – a contention which its extensive use in the Cyprus dispute amply bears out.

NOTES

1. *United Nations Charter*, Chapter VI, Article 33.
2. See *UN Doc.* S/10664, 26 May 1972, pp. 15-16, and Secretary-General's aidememoir (S/10401), 18 October 1971, Chap. V.
3. See *UN Doc.* S/5169, 25 May 1962.
4. Indar Jit Rikhye, Peace-making, Non-Violence and Truth, *International Peace Academy Reports* no. 3, 3 June 1973, p. 8.
5. See Security Council debates (S/PV.763), 23 January 1959, p. 22.
6. Ibid.
7. See *UN Doc.* S/1791, 15 September 1950, para. 99.
8. Carl M Stevens, *Strategy and Collective Bargaining Negotiations*, New York: McGraw-Hill, 1963, p. 130.
9. M. Barkun, Conflict Resolution through Implicit Mediation, *Journal of Conflict Resolution*, 8, 1964, pp. 121-30.
10. The distinction made between compromise and genuine solution is relevant in this regard; see H. A. Shepard, Responses to Situations of Competition and Conflict in Elise Boulding (ed.), *Conflict Management in Organisations*, Ann Arbor: University of Michigan Press, 1961, pp. 33-41.
11. *Official Records of the Security Council, Second Year*, agenda item 99 (document S/597), 3 November 1947, p. 2603.
12. *UN Doc.* S/651, 17 January 1948.
13. See *UN Docs.* S/7221, 24 March 1966, for provisions of the 'Tashkent Declaration', and S/7231, letter of 1 April 1966, from Pakistan; see also *Yearbook of the United Nations*, 1966, pp. 164-6.
14. See, *passim*, T. W. Adams, and A. J. Cottrell, *Cyprus Between East and West*, Baltimore: Johns Hopkins University Press, 1968; and Philip Windsor, *NATO and the Cyprus Crisis*, London: Adelphi Papers, no. 14, 1964.

15. See Edward Philip Levine, *The Mediation of International Disputes*, Ph.D. thesis, Yale University, 1971, pp. 272-5.
16. See Roger Fisher, 'Fractioning Conflict', *International Conflict and Behavioural Sciences: The Craigville Papers*, New York: Basic Books, 1964, pp 91-109.
17. This may mean that they see advantageous objectives accruing from non-resolution. See Fred Charles Ikle and Nathan Leites, 'Political Negotiation as a process of Modifying Utilities', *Journal of Conflict Resolution*, 6 no. 1, March 1962, pp. 19-28.
18. Ibid.
19. K. H. Tuncliff, 'The United Nations and the Mediation of International Conflict', Ph.D. thesis, University of Iowa, August 1984, pp. 332-4.
20. See United Nations Press Release SG/SM/1747, 12 September 1972; Press Releases NV/318 (renumbered later as NV/319) 13 October 1972, and NV/320, 20 October 1972; *Official Records of the General Assembly, Twenty-seventh Session* (A/8794) 27 September 1972, and *Twenty-seventh Session, General Committee*, 203-206th meetings (GA/4618-4622), 28 September 1972.
21. See *UN Doc*. S/2017/Rev.1, 30 March 1951; *Official Records of the Security Council, Sixth Year*, supplement for January-March 1951, para. 6, and 532nd meeting (S/PV/532), 21 February 1951.
22. *Official Records of the Security Council, Twentieth Year*, supplement for January-March 1965 (S/6253), para. 130.
23. *Official Records of the Security Council*, 1965 (S/66/47), pp. 233-4; also document S/6683, 16 September 1965, pp. 295-305.
24. Ibid., 3 September 1965 (S/6651), p. 240.
25. See *Official Records of the Security Council, Third Year*, supplement no. 2 (S/676), pp. 10-19.
26. See *Repertory of Practice of United Nations Organs*, vol. 1, paras 221-9; supplement no. 1, vol. 1, paras. 152-155; supplement no. 3, vol. 1, paras. 104-131.
27. See United Nations Press Releases SG/SM/1566-SC/3259, 27 October 1971, and note no. 3703, 28 October 1971 – communications issued on behalf of the Secretary-General and reply from the Prime Minister of India, 16 November 1971 (India Press Release no. 263/71, 17 November 1971).
28. *Official Records of the Security Council*, 181st meeting, agenda item 74, 12 August 1947, p. 1940.
29. See, in this regard, *Official Records of the Security Council*, Eighth Year, supplement no. 1 (S/2967), 1953, p. 23; also the report of Gunnar Jarring on India-Pakistan question (S/3821), 29 April 1957.
30. *UN Doc*. S/6253 and Corr.1, 26 March 1965.
31. *UN Doc*. A/90001/Add.1, 23 August 1973, p. 5.

2

THE ORIGINS OF THE CYPRUS PROBLEM FROM INDEPENDENCE TO 1964

The Independence Constitution as a basis for the sovereign state of Cyprus

The long-standing aspirations of the Greek Cypriots to achieve *Enosis* (union with Greece) were aborted with the birth of the Cyprus Republic. On 11 February 1959, in Zurich, after seven days of tough negotiations, an agreement was reached between Greece and Turkey for the establishment of the sovereign state of Cyprus. Later the agreement was accepted by the United Kingdom, Archbishop Makarios and the leader of the Turkish Cypriots, Dr Fasil Küchük. There was a Draft Treaty concerning the establishment of the Republic of Cyprus; the Draft Treaty of Guarantee between the UK, Greece, Turkey and the Republic of Cyprus; the Draft Treaty of Alliance between the Republic of Cyprus, Greece and Turkey; and finally a Gentlemen's Agreement between the Greek Premier, Karamanlis, and his Turkish counterpart, Menderes, supplemented by a Protocol. In retrospect, the independence of Cyprus was not a surprise. The post-war period had proved to be the age of nationalism and the independence of almost all the colonies: Cyprus was one among many.

There had been a background of violent nationalism in Cyprus since 1955. The organised violence conducted by the then illegal organisation EOKA,[1] combined with the diplomatic efforts of Greece, had paved the way to the establishment of the Cyprus Republic. The precedent for violent struggle for achieving *Enosis* in Cyprus had been set in 1931 when Government House (the governor's residence) was burned down as a demonstration of will to realise union with Greece. After the Second World War and the introduction of the Truman Doctrine, the aspiration for self-determination once again began to surface in Cyprus. Attempts were made to apply pressure on the British government to relinquish its sovereignty over Cyprus. Violence and diplomacy, both inspired by nationalism, were employed by the Greek Cypriots, who form the majority, towards their stated aim: *Enosis*. For them, independence was only a compromise solution and, as will be shown later, they accepted it instead of *Enosis* only because their charismatic leader, Archbishop Makarios, had done so. 'If anybody else had come back home with independence instead of Enosis,' as one prominent politician in Cyprus put it, 'he would have been chased out of the island.'[2] Some Turkish and Turkish-Cypriot scholars argue that *Enosis* is the very root of the Cyprus problem;[3] it was, after all, the prime motivating factor in the uprising of the Greek Cypriots. And it was the prospect of *Enosis*, according to Turkey and the Turkish-Cypriot leadership, which in the end alarmed the Turks of Cyprus and led to the differences that resulted in violence and tragedy.[4] Although it may be doubted whether *Enosis* was the sole cause of the sufferings in Cyprus, nonetheless a clear understanding of the concept is important for the study of the Cyprus conflict.

The population of Cyprus consists of approximately 80 per cent Greek Cypriots and 18 per cent Turkish Cypriots. The remaining 2 per cent comprises Armenians, Maronites and others. Traditionally, the two main communities in Cyprus enjoyed a state of amicable relations: historical records before 1955 indicate that they did not feel threatened by one another, and despite symbolic and important separations in their traditions and customs, there was a degree of cooperation and social intercourse between them. One report states that in some parts of Cyprus Greeks and the Turks sat in the same coffee shop together.[5] To understand the significance of this, one has to appreciate the importance of coffee shops in Cyprus as a focal point of belonging, loyalty and friendship. Underlying this amicable state of affairs, however, were two main differences – of religion and language. Greek Cypriots spoke Greek and were of Greek Orthodox denomination, whereas Turkish Cypriots spoke Turkish and practiced Islam. These differences made the two communities in Cyprus vulnerable to the influence of their mother-countries, Greece and Turkey. As a result, in the wake of Cypriot independence, the old rivalries and enmity between the Ottomans and the Greeks found an avenue to manifest themselves anew. This naturally led to an enlargement of the Cyprus issue to involve the two mother-countries which, as will be seen later, afforded Cyprus a significance out of proportion to its size or population.

In 1950 the young and newly-elected Archbishop of Cyprus, Makarios III, with the help of AKEL,[6] the Communist Party of Cyprus, arranged for a plebiscite among Greek Cypriots in order to test the popularity of *Enosis* on the island. The result was 92 per cent in favour. Subsequently Makarios, with the backing of the Greek Cypriots, started a campaign to achieve *Enosis* for Cyprus. In 1954 he took an oath to serve only for the achievement of *Enosis* and to campaign until it was attained[7] suggesting that he viewed it as an attainable goal.

There were two main concerns with regard to *Enosis*: the position of Turkish Cypriots and the position of the British government. The former had held a demonstration in the early 1950s against *Enosis*, and the latter had expressed unwillingness to discuss Cyprus at all. The famous 'never' of Henry Hopkinson, a minister at the Colonial Office, was evidence of Britain's position. On 28 July 1954, he told the House of Commons,

> It was always understood and agreed that there were certain territories in the Commonwealth which, because of their particular circumstances, could 'never' expect to be fully independent.[8]

However, on two occasions in the past Britain had offered Cyprus to Greece in return for its cooperation[9] and on both Greece had declined. So, it was not unreasonable for Makarios to assume that Britain would eventually be prepared to grant *Enosis* to Cyprus. The overwhelming numerical superiority of the Greek Cypriots was thought to be good enough, in every respect, to counter the opposition of the Turkish Cypriots.

It was in pursuit of *Enosis* that EOKA was formed under the military leadership of a Greek general of Cypriot origin, George Grivas. EOKA started a violent campaign, which had counter-productive repercussions. In the absence of a well-developed Cypriot nationalism, the appearance of an organised, radical and Greek-oriented organisation aiming at the unification of Cyprus with Greece encouraged Turkish Cypriots to cling to their traditional roots and assert their Turkishness against what seemed to them an assault by the Greek nationalism in Cyprus. The tripartite conference of 1955 in London between Britain, Greece and Turkey on the Cyprus issue achieved little in the way of coming to an acceptable solution between Greece and Turkey.

The more EOKA extended its influence over the various segments of the Greek-Cypriot community, the more Turkish identity and culture became entrenched in the minds of Turkish Cypriots, who subsequently formed a parallel institution, TMT.[10] Moreover, Turkish Cypriots started to demand partition of the island between Greece and Turkey if Britain were to relinquish its sovereignty.[11] Greek and Turkish nationalism in Cyprus now became engaged in a violent battle through EOKA and TMT. The recruitment by Britain of Turkish Cypriots as members of the auxiliary police force to combat EOKA activists merely polarised the positions of the two communities. Intercommunal violence began to spread.

In 1956, Makarios was exiled by the British administration to the Seychelles (then still a British colony), but released in the following year. From then until independence the degree of Makarios's control of events in Cyprus cannot be established clearly. He took residence in Athens after his release and tried to persuade the Greek government to apply more pressure on Britain by all possible means towards the achievement of *Enosis*.

By 1959 two factors called for urgent action on Cyprus. One was that internationalisation of the problem meant possible involvement of the Soviet Union – a worrying prospect for the West, particularly the United States. The second was the increasing number of killings in Cyprus; the actual number is disputed but is agreed to have reached at least hundreds. The British Government had frequently attempted to make peace but without success. However, after much contention and an initial agreement in Zurich, a final settlement was reached between Turkey and Greece on 19 February 1959 at Lancaster House in London. Makarios, despite earlier opposition, signed the Agreements along with the Turkish-Cypriot leader, Dr Küchük. The London Agreements included nine documents, of which the most significant were the Draft Treaty concerning the Establishment of the Republic of Cyprus; the Draft Treaty of Guarantee between Britain, Greece, Turkey and the Republic of Cyprus; the Draft Treaty of Alliance between the Republic of Cyprus, Greece and Turkey; and a 'Gentlemen's Agreement' between Karamanlis and Menderes supplemented by a protocol.

An independence constitution set out how the new republic was to function. The formation of the legislative, judicial and executive powers was designed to reflect the bicommunal nature of the Cypriot population. The House of Representatives was to have thirty-five Greek and fifteen Turkish members, elected by the Greek and Turkish communities respectively. For any bill to become law, a separate majority of the representatives of both communities was required. The cabinet, civil service and judiciary were to consist of, and employ, Greek Cypriots and Turkish Cypriots in a 70:30 ratio; in the armed forces the ratio was to 60:40. The separate municipalities, which had begun functioning *de facto* in the major cities since 1958, were now to be legitimised. Two separate communal chambers were to exercise legislative and administrative power on religious, educational and cultural matters. They were also to regulate matters of personal status including the imposition of taxes to finance institutions controlled by each community.

As for the Treaty of Guarantee, Britain, Greece and Turkey undertook to guarantee the independence, territorial integrity, security and constitutional structure of the Republic. All three would have the right to secure the observance of all provisions of the treaty. In case of a breach of a provision, when concerted action proved impossible each of the guarantor powers reserved the right to act 'with the sole aim of re-establishing the state of affairs created by the present Treaty' (Art. IV). The three states would guarantee the two main sovereign bases, as well as other small bases, granted to Britain. Union with any other state, and partition, were prohibited (Art. II). The terms of the Treaty of Alliance between Cyprus, Greece and Turkey stated that the three states would cooperate and consult for their defence and protect the territorial integrity of the Republic, among other means by creating a tripartite headquarters, and by stationing a 950-man Greek and a 650-man Turkish contingent on the island. Lastly, the Gentlemen's Agreement asked for the promotion of Cyprus's participation in NATO by Greece and Turkey, and for the mother states to seek to persuade the president and the vice-president of the Republic to outlaw the Communist Party. It also called for a general amnesty to be proclaimed soon after the signing of the treaties.

Independence for Cyprus represented a 'compromise between the Greek demand for union with Greece and the Turkish counter-demand for partition between Greece and Turkey'.[13] The constitution of the new republic was viewed differently by the two communities. The Greek Cypriots saw it as an unfair framework; as put by Markides:

> Very few Greek Cypriots, including both supporters and opponents of Makarios, accepted the constitution as legitimate: [...] Most importantly the Greeks felt that the constitution discriminated against them – the majority comprising 80 percent of the population – in favour of the Turkish minority, which composed only 18 percent of the population.[14]

Turkish Cypriots, however, asserted that they should not be viewed by others as a minority but rather as a community in Cyprus.[15] As such, they claimed, Greek Cypriots' concern over the constitution was unjustified and unnecessary. There was also an extremist element among Turkish Cypriots, which saw Cyprus as an extension of Turkey and an association called 'Cyprus is a Turkish Party' had been established which nurtured radical Turkish thinking.[16] Although by and large such radical elements were a minority in the Turkish Cypriot community, their existence nonetheless left the Greek Cypriots with an impression which was not conducive to a smooth and peaceable relationship, particularly in the context of the power-sharing called for by the independence constitution.

The more important aspect of the constitution concerned its bicommunal nature. To all intents and purposes it allowed each community to operate as a distinct group, but by so doing it led to the institutionalisation of communal differences, preventing what it had initially set out to do: namely, reintegrate the two communities. Because of the mistrust that had already developed between them in the years immediately preceding independence, this further reinforced their differences. With hindsight this can clearly be seen as an inherent weakness. Makarios proposed certain changes to the constitution immediately before independence, but they were not accepted. Having finally accepted the Treaties as they stood, he returned home in triumph on 1 March 1959.

On 13 December 1959, he was elected president by the Greek Cypriot community, with 67 per cent of the votes. On 16 August 1960 he, Vice-President Küchük and the council of ministers swore an oath of loyalty to the sovereign state of Cyprus in the House of Representatives. Cyprus became independent on that day.

The new Republic of Cyprus was born in a sympathetic international climate, in which independence was perceived to be a political necessity for every country in the world. However, independence did not mean the end of the *Enosis* idea for every Greek Cypriot. Makarios himself, as will be seen later, had not totally abandoned it, and his commitment to the constitution was subject to some doubt. Only a month before the declaration of independence, he had said in a public speech:

> The Agreements do not form the goal. They are the present and not the future. The Greek Cypriot people will continue their national cause and shape their future in accordance with their will. The Zurich and London Agreements have a number of positive elements but also negative ones, and the Greeks will work to take advantage of the positive elements and get rid of the negative ones.[17]

The position of Makarios was a curious one: on the one hand, he was legally and internationally obliged to work under the constitution but, on the other hand, he was viewed by the Greek Cypriots as their leader (ethnarch) and therefore charged by them with achieving *Enosis.* Although it is difficult to establish to what degree the Greek Cypriots actually supported *Enosis* after the independence of Cyprus, it is clear that the idea had not been buried and still enjoyed considerable support. Hence Makarios had a contradictory role. To work for the achievement of *Enosis* could be seen as directly at variance with his role as president. He had to strike a balance between these two goals, and try to appease the right-wing elements in the Greek-Cypriot community, who were diehard *Enosists*: to achieve this, he was forced to grant concessions to the radicals, e.g. by appointing Polycarpos Yorgadjis as Minister of the Interior. Makarios's faith in the Cypriot constitution, however great or little it may have been in the early months of independence, was almost non-existent after the first year of the republic.[18] Whether or not he was truly working towards the achievement of *Enosis* after independence is a different matter and cannot be established unequivocally.

The Turkish Cypriots were pleased with the constitution, but their leader Küchük suspected the *bona fides* of Makarios and his seven ministers in the cabinet. Perhaps one of the reasons for this scepticism was the fact that Makarios never took Küchük, despite his position as, vice-president, into his confidence over his dilemma with the *Enosists.*[19] Makarios was an intelligent and charismatic man who was alleged to know one-third of the Greek-Cypriot population by their first names.

Internationally, the Cyprus republic was identified with him as president and national leader. Considering Makarios's standing at home and abroad, the promotion of some EOKA members in the government, and the distance between Makarios and Küchük, there was no incentive on the part of Turkish Cypriots to reintegrate with their Greek counterparts. On the contrary, their suspicions kept Turkish Cypriots alert and led to close ties being fastened with Turkey.

After independence intercommunal differences started to manifest in two important issues. One was Makarios's refusal to recruit sufficient Turks to maintain the 70:30 ratio in the civil service, based on the premise that there were not enough educated Turkish Cypriots to fill the vacant posts. The second contentious issue was the question of separate municipalities. According to the constitution, each community was to have its own municipal administration which, according to Greek Cypriots, was divisive, costly and unnecessary. Separate municipalities in the five major towns – Nicosia, Paphos, Famagusta, Limmassol and Larnaka – as required by the constitution, would have interrupted the functioning of the municipal powers, as these towns were already functioning smoothly under one united municipal administration. Although the Greek Cypriots may have had a point here, they failed to convince the Turkish Cypriots, for whom the civil service issue and the question of municipalities became a 'touch-stone for the good faith of Greek Cypriots'.[20] The army was another contentious issue, with the president seeking to have one national army and the vice-president preferring a separate Turkish-Cypriot contingent.

These disputes increased mistrust and led to the Turkish Cypriots starting to impede the routine procedures of the government necessary for the functioning of the state. The first incident occurred in the spring of 1961, when the Turkish Cypriot members of the House of Representatives, in retaliation for the civil service dispute, refused to support an extension of the country's tax laws. This led to Makarios using presidential decree for the collection of taxes – which had not been provided for in the constitution. In 1963 the constitutional court declared the decree unconstitutional. Differences also began to show within the structure of the state. In 1963 the Council of Ministers voted to establish an army in which soldiers from the two communities would be integrated, but Küchük vetoed this decision on the ground that an integrated army would be unable to function. As a result, Makarios announced that he would not establish an army at all.[21]

The only institutionalised political party in Cyprus at the time, the Communist Party AKEL, enjoyed the support of some 30 per cent of Greek Cypriots, including important elements in the trade unions. The party had aligned itself with Makarios and in return he had offered it five seats in the Parliament. The alliance carried certain benefits for both sides, since there were common elements that bound them: their common opposition to any participation by Cyprus in NATO and their full support for Cyprus' membership of the Non-Aligned movement.

The Makarios-AKEL alliance also hold an advantage for Turkish Cypriots, which emanated from the anti-*Enosis* stance of AKEL. The party's opposition to the inclusion of Cyprus in the Western camp naturally allayed some of the fears of Turkish Cypriots concerning *Enosis*. A striking advantage for Küchük was the united front of Turkish Cypriots against the Greek Cypriots in all political battles. Greek Cypriots did not enjoy such a unity, and differences of opinion among them showed very openly, since their community enjoyed greater democracy.

On 30 November 1963 Makarios proposed thirteen points as a means of attaining a smoother functioning of the state machinery. The proposals were as follows:[22]

1. The right of veto of the president and the vice-president of the republic to be abolished.
2. The vice-president of the republic to deputise for or replace the president of the republic in case of his temporary absence or incapacity to perform his duties. In consequence, therefore, all the constitutional provisions in respect of joint action by the president and the vice-president of the republic to be modified accordingly.
3. The Greek president of the House of Representatives and its Turkish vice-president to be elected by the House as a whole and not as at present the president by the Greek Members of the House and the vice-president by the Turkish Members of the House.
4. The vice-president of the House of Representatives to deputise for or replace the president of the House in case of his temporary absence or incapacity to perform his duties.
5. The constitutional provisions regarding a separate majority for enactment of laws by the House of Representatives to be abolished.
6. The constitutional provision regarding the establishment of separate municipalities in the five main towns to be abolished. Provision should be made so that:

(a) The municipal council in each of the aforesaid five towns shall consist of Greek and Turkish councillors in proportion to the number of the Greek and Turkish inhabitants of such town by whom they shall be elected respectively.
(b) In the budget of each of such aforesaid towns, after deducting any expenditure required for common services, a percentage of the balance proportionate to the number of the Turkish inhabitants of such town shall be earmarked and disposed of in accordance with the wishes of the Turkish councillors.

7. The constitutional provision regarding courts consisting of Greek judges to try Greeks and of Turkish judges to try Turks and of mixed courts consisting of Greek and Turkish judges to try cases where the litigants are Greeks and Turks to be abolished.

8. The division of the security forces into police and gendarmerie to be abolished, (provision to be made in case the head of the police is a Greek the deputy head to be a Turk and vice versa).
9. The numerical strength of the security forces and of the army to be determined by law and not by agreement between the president and the vice-president of the republic.
10. The proportion of the participation of Greek and Turkish Cypriots in the composition of the public service and of the forces of the Republic, i.e. the police and the army, to be modified in proportion to the ratio of the population of Greek and Turkish Cypriots.
11. The number of the members of the Public Service Commission to be reduced from ten to either five or seven.
12. All the decisions of the Public Service Commission to be taken by simple majority. If there is allegation of discrimination on the unanimous request either of the Greek or of the Turkish members of the Commission, its Chairman to be bound to refer the matter to the Supreme Constitutional Court.
13. The Greek Communal Chamber to be abolished.

Unsurprisingly, these proposals were strongly opposed by the Turkish Cypriot leaders and Turkey, giving rise to the possibility of Turkish military intervention. They were also opposed by the Greek government and a number of Greek Cypriot intellectuals.[23] Though the proposals may have seemed promising, and may have been well intended, they were ill-timed and lacked sufficient diplomatic and psychological preparation.[24] They sparked off a wave of violence on the island, resurrecting the Cyprus problem in the international community, and in a very acute manner.

The 1963-4 Crisis

It is beyond the scope of this study to describe the events of the 1963-4 crisis in detail. Since independence, both communities had been arming themselves to be ready for a possible conflict[25] and this had intensified in the last quarter of 1963. The immediate cause of the conflict occurred on 20 December 1963, when a few Turkish Cypriot civilians refused to obey the orders of Greek Cypriot police officers. An argument followed and during the confrontation, which had attracted a huge crowd, shots were heard and a few people died. On the following day the violence spread to the whole of Nicosia. Killings started, and intercommunal relations between Greek and Turkish Cypriots became much worse. A Christmas Eve peace-call by the leaders of both communities did not stop the fighting.

The clear negative response by the two communities to their leaders' pledge to put an end to the violence demonstrated the severity of the situation. The numerical superiority of the Greek Cypriots gave them the upper hand in the physical confrontations; nonetheless, the Turkish

Cypriots managed to exert considerable influence on the events that followed. All Turkish state employees left their positions and, along with the rest of Turkish Cypriots, under the direct control of their leader, began to effect the geographical separation of the communities by choosing to go into enclaves and isolate themselves from the Greek Cypriots. Any Turkish Cypriot associating with any Greek Cypriot at this time would have been taking a serious risk. This self-imposed isolation is believed by some to have been part of a premeditated plot to prove to the world that the Greeks and Turks of Cyprus could not live side by side under a unitary government.

Turkey warned the Cyprus government, which by then was dominated by Greek Cypriots, of its grave concern over the crisis. In late December 1963 it sent military jets over Cyprus in an attempt to pressurise the Greek Cypriots. Turkey seemed to be preparing to take military action, but was deterred by a strong letter from the US President Lyndon Johnson. At a five-party conference in London, the idea of a NATO peacekeeping force was introduced, but was rejected by Makarios. The backing of the Soviet premier Nikita Khrushchev made Makarios more confident in his stand against any NATO military presence on the island. The plan of US Secretary of State Dean Acheson – outlined in the following pages – was also vetoed by Makarios. Subsequently, early in 1964, Makarios took the issue to the United Nations.

On 4 March, the Security Council passed Resolution 186, authorising the dispatch of a UN peacekeeping force to the island. A mediator was also appointed to try to bring about a compromise solution to the problem. The sudden death on 9 September of the Finnish mediator Sakari Tuomioja led to the appointment of Dr Galo Plaza, who produced a full report which is discussed in the next chapter.

The 1963-4 crisis had some significant implications. First, it showed the determination of Makarios to go ahead with the changes in the constitution despite the possiblity of a Turkish military intervention, and despite the threat of a serious rift which could follow between the two communities. There was no reason to believe that the Turkish Cypriots, or Turkey, had the slightest intention of agreeing to Makarios's proposals; on the contrary, there was every indication that they would have not accepted any change in the *status quo*.[26] It may be supposed either that Makarios felt prepared for any form of opposition from the Turks, military or otherwise, or that he naively believed his proposed changes would eventually come into force without much disruption. As state President, as leader of the majority of the population and as leader of the independence struggle he considered himself entitled by right to propose changes and – in the event of a Turkish Cypriot withdrawal from the government – to go ahead with them. He is quoted by Dimitrios Bitsios as saying: 'I have no reason to appeal to the United Nations.

I am the head of state and I shall implement my decisions. Let those who disagree appeal to the United Nations, and then we shall see....'[27]

Makarios had not agreed with some of terms of the constitution from the beginning, and had no role in the process of devising it. He expressed his feelings about the constitution in 1964:

> At the Conference of Lancaster House in February, 1959, which I was invited to attend as the leader of the Greek Cypriots, I raised a number of objections and expressed strong misgivings regarding certain provisions of the Agreements arrived at in Zurich between the Greek and the Turkish Governments and adopted by the British Government. I tried very hard to bring about the change of at least some provisions of that Agreement. I failed, however, in that effort and I was faced with dilemma either of signing the Agreement as it stood or of rejecting it with all the grave consequences which would have ensued. In the circumstances I had no alternative but to sign the Agreement. This was the course dictated to me by necessity.[28]

Another important implication of the 1963-4 crisis was the readiness of the Turkish Cypriots in such circumstances to assert themselves as a recognisable force. This indicated some sort of organisation which could not have been in operation without the help of Turkey. Many Turkish military officers travelled back and forth between Ankara and Nicosia in the 1960-3 period. The capture by Turkish Cypriots of the Nicosia-Kyrenia road towards the end of 1963 was a planned military action aimed at maintaining access to the capital from the north in case Turkey decided to launch a military operation against its soft underbelly – Cyprus. Whether they anticipated the crisis or merely felt that they could not afford to be unprepared for this eventuality is not clear.

The crisis of 1963 also highlighted the weak points of the constitution. It is true that if Makarios had not advanced his proposals for thirteen amendments, it would probably not have occurred, but the proposals were more of a catalyst than the underlying cause, which was the deep mistrust between the two communities, particularly between their leaders. As the head of state Makarios had a right to propose amendments to the constitution; in fact, any high-ranking official or state personality could have done so or made counter-proposals. The mere fact of Makarios proposing changes need not have led to intercommunal violence had there not already been an underlying cause for the conflict, nor is there any reason to believe that the conflict would not have occurred at some near future date even if Makarios had complied with every article of the constitution. The issue of separate municipalities was a prime example of constitutional requirements conflicting with the needs of an efficient administration, and the mere operation of this arrangement could have acted as an immediate cause of conflict. The implementation of certain other constitutional provisions, e.g. on the civil service, could also have proved troublesome and sparked off violence. A further implication of the crisis was the Cypriot people's lack of confidence in the machinery of their government: had it been efficient it should have been able to resolve its own problems without provoking intercommunal violence.

As the violence continued, the intercommunal mistrust deepened. In the Mansoura area of Paphos many Turkish Cypriots – although Greek Cypriots claim that the Turkish Cypriots started the incident themselves – were subjected to brutality, and many were killed or seriously injured. The EOKA leader Grivas had by now been sent back to Nicosia from Greece as the only man able to gather all the Greek Cypriot fighters under a military command. Makarios established the Greek Cypriot National Guard as Turkish fighter planes started bombing Greek Cypriots. Following diplomatic representation at the UN, the killings in Mansoura and the air attacks stopped. However, the problem of Cyprus – now no longer a colony but a sovereign state – had reappeared and was to have disturbing international repercussions.

Outside powers and Cyprus till 1964

The United Kingdom. Britain's great wealth and military power in the nineteenth century and the first half of the twentieth resulted in its gaining possession and control over many overseas territories. However, the consequences of the two world wars and the spread of nationalist aspirations throughout the colonies led to massive changes in the British Empire and the relinquishment of sovereignty over most colonies. The appearance of the United States and the Soviet Union as the superpowers of the post-Second World War era – both of them ideologically opposed to colonialism – emphasised the need for Britain to readjust to a changing world.

Cyprus had been ruled by the British Empire since 1878. On 24 July 1923, by the Treaty of Lausanne, Turkey gave up all its rights over the island and Cyprus became a British colony. The importance of Cyprus to the interests of the United Kingdom has varied in recent times. At the 1912-13 conference in London over the Balkan crisis, Lloyd George offered *Enosis* to the Greek Prime Minister, Venizelos, in return for a British base at Argostoli or Cephallonia.[29] In 1915 *Enosis* was again offered in return for Greek cooperation in the war. On both occasions that offer was turned down, so at this time Cyprus could not have seemed – to either party – a great asset. During the Second World War Cyprus was offered to Greece by Germany in return for neutrality in the conflict but again the offer was rejected.

The diplomatic pressures on Britain to emancipate all its colonies, including Cyprus, started on 14 August 1941 with the Atlantic Charter, signed by the British prime minister Winston Churchill and the US President Franklin D. Roosevelt. The Charter required, inter alia, the emancipation of all colonies, and when President Truman took office in 1945 he called for its speedy implementation. Having just rid itself of the dangers of a communist takeover with British and American help, Greece felt encouraged by the international climate to pursue the case for unification with Cyprus. However, despite its awareness of the Greek position, Britain refused to admit that there was such a 'Cyprus problem', preferring to cling to the *status quo* for the time being. Dimitrios Bitsios, a Greek official who was actively involved in the diplomatic aspects of the problem, quotes King George VI as saying to the Greek ambassador in London in 1951: 'Yes, about Cyprus. I am aware of your démarche. Tell your people in Athens that it is preferable for all of us to leave things as they are for the time being. It is a matter of common security.'[30]

In September 1953 the British foreign secretary, Anthony Eden, repeated the same message in Athens to the Greek prime minister, Field-Marshal Papagos. Britain's stubborn refusal to deal with the question of Cyprus was particularly incomprehensible to the Greeks and it is sometimes suggested that the Colonial Office was deliberately delaying the handling of the problem until Turkey could be sufficiently motivated to take part in any forthcoming negotiations. In 1955 the British foreign secretary in Eden's government formed that year, Harold Macmillan, invited Greece and Turkey to London for discussions on Cyprus. Only a year earlier, the then colonial secretary, Henry Hopkinson, had made his declaration in the House of Commons that certain colonies – he was clearly alluding to Cyprus[31] – could never expect to be fully independent. The change in British policy between 1954 and 1959 is sometimes attributed to the changes of government in Britain. 'The replacement of Eden by Macmillan as prime minister in the aftermath of the Suez Canal crisis began the process that led to the 1959 settlement.'[32]

At a conference convened on 30 June 1955 at Lancaster House in London, Turkey and Greece found themselves in opposing positions over Cyprus. It is sometimes suggested that this tripartite conference was an attempt by Britain to put the Greeks and the Turks at loggerheads,[33] but Greece and Turkey, with their long history of conflict, could not avoid being in conflict over the issue. It may be argued with hindsight that Britain might have diminished the rivalry by giving greater encouragement to the integration of the two communities on the island.[34] Be that as it may, the 1955 conference did not achieve a compromise over Cyprus, and thereafter tension increased.

With the outbreak of the Suez crisis in 1956 the significance of

Cyprus was suddenly enhanced. Its strategic location making it the key to Western Asia began to be more fully appreciated: with good weather throughout the year, it was highly suitable for military training, and also provided a convenient base for British intelligence to monitor the activities of the states in the region, particularly the Soviet Union. The latter was of particular significance to NATO at the time in the light of the intense Cold War competition and the accompanying build-up of the Soviet Union's armed forces. Its strategic significance aside, Britain's concern over Cyprus resulted from two other important considerations: the effect on other British colonies, particularly Malta, of granting any self-rule, sometimes referred to as the 'domino effect', and its intense desire not to upset the Muslim world. Some argue that this last consideration influenced the British government's attitude to Turkey. This view finds support in a remark made by Alan Lennox-Boyd, the Secretary of State for the Colonies, in the House of Commons on 15 July 1957:

> If the Turks have fears, are these fears not fostered by the Archbishop's attempt to prevent their having a full say in their own future, not only as people who are an important minority but as people whose mother-land is only forty miles away, while the main-land of Greece is many hundreds of miles away?[35]

Lennox-Boyd had already clearly stated on 19 December 1956 that if the principle of self-determination was to be applied in Cyprus, it would be applied to both communities separately.[36] In other words, partition would be the automatic result of self-determination, if that was what the Greeks wanted.

At home, the British Conservative government of the time was being heavily criticised by the Labour Party and others for its Cyprus policy. Harold Nicolson wrote in his diary that on 29 October 1956, 'Eden and Selwyn Lloyd made revoltingly unctuous statements in the House about Hungary. When people rise against foreign oppression they are hailed as patriots and heroes; but the Greeks whom we are shooting and hanging in Cyprus are dismissed as terrorists. What cant!'[37]

The possibility of granting self-determination to the whole of Cyprus on a majority-minority basis, which would have inevitably have led to *Enosis*, was out of the question. Turkey was too important a country to be ignored: its strategic significance and membership of NATO made it an indispensable ally. On the other hand, separate self-determination for both communities, though not wholly rejected by Greece, was totally unacceptable to Makarios. Britain was looking for a solution that could accommodate its interests and at the same time keep the belligerent parties satisfied.

Meanwhile Sir Hugh Foot (later Lord Caradon) had replaced Field-

Marshal Harding as governor of Cyprus. This was viewed by Greeks and Greek Cypriots as an encouraging sign and it was during his governorship that the British Prime Minister, Harold Macmillan, came up with a formula to resolve the Cyprus problem. His plan for the administration of the island, announced in June 1958, required consultation between the Cyprus governor and special representatives of Greece and Turkey who would enjoy equal status. For Makarios this plan was tantamount to disaster; he could not tolerate the involvement of Turkey in the administration of Cyprus. Later in 1958 Barbara Castle, then chairman of the Labour Party, came to an agreement with Makarios whereby *Enosis* and partition would be excluded from any settlement by a future Labour government and Cyprus would be an independent state and part of the Commonwealth. As it turned out, the Agreement reached in 1960 was not much different. Britain would obtain sovereign military bases on the island at Akrotiri and Dhekelia. The 1960 Agreement paved way for the establishment of the independent sovereign state of Cyprus.

Despite all the ups and downs, the 1960 Agreements contained the elements to satisfy the main concerns of Britain – the exclusion of *Enosis* and partition. Britain had also managed to maintain its interests by keeping the Sovereign Bases while relieving itself of troubled intercommunal relations between the Greek and Turkish Cypriots.

The breakdown of the Republic in 1963 did not damage Britain's interests in any way. However, its role, in the control and the containment of the crisis is somewhat unclear. The thirteen points proposed by Makarios were, according to Kyrris, encouraged by Britain[38] although it had no reason to believe that such proposals would be welcomed by Turkey. Also, the unexplained withdrawal of Lieutenant Martin Packard from his successful mediatory post in Nicosia, when a settlement of the conflict was in prospect, has never been explained by Britain.[39] At any rate, after the crisis both mother-countries, Greece and Turkey, looked to Britain to try to arrange a peaceful settlement to the crisis. The intervention of British troops on 29 December 1963 came in time to establish the so called 'Green Line' between the two communities in Nicosia. A new conference convened in London between 15 January and 10 February 1964 failed to achieve an agreement, and once again the situation seemed deadlocked.

Greece. After the War of Independence in the early nineteenth century, which led to the establishment of the modern Greek state, Hellenism found new strength among the Greeks. Greek Cypriots shared this reawakened pride in their heritage, and the idea of *Enosis* was propounded as an inevitable outcome of the strong emotional links between Greece and the Greek Cypriots. However, in the twentieth century the attitude of Greece towards *Enosis* fluctuated. After the First World War the Greek premier, Venizelos, dissuaded the Greek delegation from asking for *Enosis* at the Versailles peace conference, because he needed British help in his plans for Asia Minor. The desire of the Greek Cypriots for *Enosis* on the one hand, and the ambivalence of Greece towards it on the other, are summarised by Tremayne: 'Cypriots are Greeks; but Greeks are not Cypriots. The two temperaments are widely different.'[40]

After the civil war in Greece (1944-9), the pursuit of *Enosis* did not cease to be a national issue and one to which Greek policy, at least officially, had to adhere, although this varied with different governments. For instance, while in the early 1950s Field-Marshal Papagos was totally pro-*Enosis*, his successor Karamanlis had different ideas. The main obstacles to Greece supporting *Enosis* whole-heartedly were put clearly by George Papandreou, Greece's interior minister, also in the early 1950s, when he told a Greek-Cypriot delegation calling for *Enosis*: 'Greece breathes with two lungs, one British and the other American, and it cannot suffocate for the sake of the Cypriot problem.'[41] Caught between *Enosists* on the one hand, and its NATO obligations on the other, Greece now promised, in exchange for *Enosis*, NATO bases not only in Cyprus but additional ones in Greece.[42] The Greek prime minister told the British ambassador: 'One would be able to say not just that Cyprus had been annexed by Greece, but Greece in its entirety had been annexed by Britain.'[43]

In 1954, in spite of Western pressure to the contrary, Greece took the Cyprus issue to the United Nations, but failed to gain support for *Enosis*. With the coming to power of Karamanlis as prime minister in 1955, Greek policy towards Cyprus, though officially unchanged, reached a turning point. Karamanlis knew well that in a conflict Turkey's superior military might would mean defeat and the surrender of Cyprus to Turkey. His stance affected the influence of Greece in Cyprus and over Makarios. He was not as active a supporter of *Enosis* as his predecessor, and this helped a distinct Cypriot consciousness to grow stronger. After his return from exile, during which Greece had withdrawn its ambassador from London in protest, Makarios was not welcomed at the airport in Athens by Karamanlis, nor was his speech broadcast on Greek television or radio.[44] In fact, the Karamanlis era proved a difficult one for the Greek Cypriots. In 1958 Makarios had proposed to the Greek government that Greece should withdraw from NATO if the Macmillan plan, referred to in the previous section, were implemented, but Karamanlis refused even to contemplate such a policy and instead pressured Makarios to accept the London-Zurich Agreements.

The acceptance of the London-Zurich Agreements by Greece put the Greek prime minister in a difficult position: he faced a censure motion, which however was eventually defeated. The military commander of EOKA, General George Grivas, expressing a general feeling in Cyprus and Greece, wrote: 'No-one in Cyprus today can approve the handling of the national question by the Karamanlis government.'[45] After the independence of Cyprus, the *Enosis* file, as far as Karamanlis was concerned, was shelved and the thirteen-point proposals put forward by Makarios in 1963 were rejected by Greece.

Following the departure from office of Karamanlis in 1963, a meeting was held between Makarios and the new Greek prime minister, George Papandreou, and this led to an agreement between them on four points. First, the Cyprus problem was to be solved by the United Nations and not by NATO. Secondly, *Enosis* was to be the ultimate aim. Thirdly, no action would be taken that might provoke Turkey to take military action against Cyprus, and some concessions would be made to the Turkish Cypriots. Finally, Greece would come to the aid of Cyprus should Turkey decide to attack the island,[46] and to give credence to this last point Greece sent around 10,000 troops to Cyprus. In addition Papandreou declared: 'A clash between Greece and Turkey would be murder, but if Turkey decides to enter the mad-house we shall not hesitate to follow her.'[47]

Overall, Greece's participation in NATO was too important a commitment to be ignored and too beneficial an alliance to be set aside and thus it played an important role in Greece's diplomatic manoeuvring. The Greek premier, for instance, stated in Parliament on 14 March 1957:

> Greece is obligated to conduct the Cyprus struggle within the boundaries of her alliance. This last point renders the Cyprus problem an issue with dramatic contradictions. There are moments during which a policy that promotes the Cyprus problem could be damaging for free Greece. On the other hand [there may be] instances during which an act that may be right for Greece becomes damaging to Cyprus.[48]

Nonetheless, the pressure of public opinion and the traditional links with Cyprus were commitments in their own right. At this time *Enosis* was a policy which the Greek government could under no circumstance abandon. The national feeling was expressed by King Constantine when he said on 31 December 1964, 'I wish our Cypriot brothers a speedy union with the mother country.'[49]

In its treatment of Cyprus, Greece expected the island to follow its direction, and for Cyprus this created difficulties. For instance, at the peak of intercommunal tension, Papandreou wrote to Makarios on 24 August 1964:

> No decision shall be taken in Cyprus that may lead directly or indirectly to hostilities without our approval. The opinion of Athens must be

final, for it is Athens that bears the responsibility of the whole of Hellenism. [...] I mean that as a result of your lifelong arduous struggles you have acquired a habit of making policy decisions alone.[50]

By 1964, then, Greece's policy towards Cyprus had precluded a confrontation with Turkey, but at the same time had not totally abandoned the idea of *Enosis*.

Turkey. The part played by Turkey in the development of events in Cyprus, both historically and in the modern era, can hardly be exaggerated. The Turks had conquered the island in 1571 and established the institution of Ethnarchy (head of the nation) as the political head of the Greek Cypriots. In 1878, after defeat by the Russians, and in fear of them, the Ottoman empire agreed to leave the administration of Cyprus to Britain in return for help in the event of a Russian military advance against it. In 1914 Britain annexed Cyprus and nine years later at the peace conference in Lausanne, Turkey renounced all claims to territories outside its boundaries, including Cyprus. Two years later Cyprus became a crown colony of Britain.

Between then and 1955, when it officially acknowledged its involvement in the Cyprus problem by accepting an invitation to the tripartite conference in London, Turkey had shown little interest in Cyprus. However, some attribute its reticence in this period to the friendly attitude of Britain towards Turkey and the Turkish Cypriots. Turkey, they argue, perceived no threat in the *status quo* before 1955, and therefore had no need to make public statements about it. However, during the London conference the Turkish foreign minister, Fatin Zorlu, expressed his government's wishes to resist *Enosis*, at any cost.[51] Soon after that, severe anti-Greek riots broke out in Istanbul, where there was still a large Greek population, with slogans against *Enosis* which the then prime minister Menderes later admitted had been instigated by the Turkish government.[52]

As *Enosis* appeared to be at the forefront of the Greek government's claim, Turkey for its part argued that Cyprus should be given back to Turkey should Britain decide to leave the island. Later, however, the Turkish government modified its view and put forward the idea of partitioning the island.

Following developments in Cyprus during the latter half of the 1950s, the idea of a paramilitary organisation to oppose EOKA was put into practice, and TMT was established. 'Cyprus is a Turkish party' was also set up by a Turkish national who came to Cyprus with the aim of centralising the political efforts of the Turkish Cypriots. It is indisputable that just as EOKA received its arms directly from Greece, TMT also received its military supplies from Turkey. On 19 October 1959 the Turkish ship *Deniz*, transporting arms and ammunition to the Turkish

Cypriots, was sunk by its crew off Kyrenia, both to escape arrest by Cypriot officials and to destroy the evidence of an arms shipment from Turkey to Cyprus.[53]

The domestic situation in Turkey was difficult during the 1950s: economic hardship was a constant source of discontent and of criticism of the government by the opposition. Deflecting attention to Cyprus served as a useful means of softening attacks on Menderes's government.

After the independence of Cyprus, Turkish officers made regular trips to Nicosia and made a thorough survey of the military positions of the Greeks. They also prepared a military wing of the Turkish Cypriots to cope with any outbreak of violence, and it was this preparation that made the Turkish Cypriots an effective force against the Greek Cypriots in December 1963. Before the outbreak of violence in 1963, Turkey had rejected Makarios's proposals even before the Turkish Cypriot leader had said anything about them.[54] This dominant position over Turkish Cypriots was something that both Turkey and the Turkish Cypriot leadership took for granted. In 1974 the leader of Turkish Cypriots, Rauf Denktash, retorted to accusations of being a 'tool in the hands of Turkey' that such remarks were absurd since he was a 'part of Turkey'.[55]

Turkey is a strategically important country in the Near East. It had joined NATO in 1952 and was therefore bound by the concerns and the interests of the alliance. Two of these concerns were particularly irritating for Turkey where Cyprus was concerned. First, Turkey could not engage in a war with Greece without endangering the alliance and secondly any easing of relations with its Soviet neighbour was viewed with anxiety by the United States. Its rift with the Soviets, which was implicit in its membership of the Western alliance, proved costly for Turkey: it was Soviet support for Cyprus in 1964 that led to a warning to the Turkish prime minister Inönü by President Johnson, deterring Turkey from taking any action against Cyprus. Nonetheless, it sent two of its jets over Cyprus in an attempt to pressurise the Greek Cypriot leadership, and on 7 and 8 August 1964 it dropped bombs, causing civilian casualties.

Turkey's attitude to Cyprus reflected two major considerations: one was its security concerns and the other its desire to protect the Turkish Cypriot community. These concerns are interrelated and inseparable, although many contend that security was the more important.[56] This view was also expressed by Turkish officials, though more subtly. A former Turkish foreign minister, Günes, said in 1980:

> 'Cyprus is a huge aircraft carrier that is anchored in the most strategic part of the Eastern Mediterranean. It keeps the whole Eastern Mediterranean under military control. It is one step off the Turkish coast and two steps from the Arab peninsula. It is like a Guardian of

the Suez Canal. Without keeping in mind the strategic importance of Cyprus...it is impossible to understand the whole Cyprus crisis.'[57]

In the light of these important considerations and its NATO obligations, Turkey faced a dilemma in 1964. Any action against Cyprus was doomed to failure as the Soviets were prepared to support the Cyprus government, and the idea of stepping aside without doing anything was perceived by Turkish policy-makers as against its interests. Thus a more conciliatory approach seemed the best option. If Greece and Turkey could somehow reach an agreement whereby Turkey's strategic interests could be secured without the need for military action or a shift in its alliances, then Cyprus and the Cypriots could also reap the benefits.

The United States. With the introduction of the Truman Doctrine in 1947, the hopes of the Greek Cypriots were raised in anticipation of American support for *Enosis*. As events developed, however, these early hopes were dashed, as the United States became aware of the likely repercussions of any encouragement for *Enosis*. The overriding feature of the global political arena at the time was the bipolarity of the Cold War, so that the security of the West necessitated careful formulation of policy. It was in this framework that the State Department took the initiative to settle the Cyprus problem.

The United States was deeply concerned that any problem within the Western family should be solved discreetly, through 'quiet diplomacy'. Any attempt to internationalise the issue would prove costly to the West, as the Soviets would undoubtedly exploit intra-Western embarrassment for propaganda purposes. So when in 1954 Greece took the issue before the UN, it received no support or sympathy from the United States. Moreover, a Greco-Turkish rift would have posed a threat to the credibility of NATO: Turkey and Greece formed its southeastern flank, and the question of Cyprus could not be allowed to bring them into military conflict with each another. This threat gave the United States an impetus to settle the problem before it could compromise the security of the West. Accordingly, it continued its efforts through NATO to promote a peaceful solution. There was added urgency in the need to avoid damaging the position of the Cyprus government: with the significant Cypriot communist party, AKEL, in the wings, a failure on the Cyprus front would risk enhancing the prospect of a communist regime in Cyprus.

It is sometimes suggested that confronted with such a potentially dangerous and delicate issue, the American policy-makers were biased towards Turkey as the more important country, and in so doing put themselves in a difficult situation. Some observers regarded both countries as equally important.[58] This tilt towards Turkey at times upset US relations with Greece, although Greek economic dependence maintained

American leverage over Greek politicians. The US government was relieved by the eventual signing of the London-Zurich Agreements, not knowing of course that this was to be only a temporary solution.

With independence, friendly relations were established between the United States and the new Republic of Cyprus. Armed conflict between Turkey and Greece having apparently receded from the Cyprus scenario, American concern at this stage was to contain AKEL. The Gentlemen's Agreement required the assistance of Greece and Turkey in persuading the Cyprus government to ban communism on the island. However, events confounded this goal: by reaching an agreement with the AKEL leaders, Makarios narrowed the gap between his government and the communists.

The outbreak of hostilities in December 1963 alarmed the United States for several reasons. First, there was the possibility of a serious rift between two NATO countries, which now looked more dangerous than hitherto. Secondly, Makarios had proved an untrustworthy ally, leading Cyprus towards the Non-Aligned countries and involving AKEL in the running of the country. Thirdly, the Cyprus issue had exposed to the world a serious internal difficulty within the Western camp. And last but not least was the spectre of Cyprus turning into a Mediterranean Cuba. Besides the urgency of averting a Greco-Turkish war, Makarios needed to be restrained: independent and powerful as he was at the time, he was seen as untrustworthy. The frustration of the United States with him grew, as time went on, as is described later.

Following a halt in the fighting of December 1963, US Secretary of State Dean Acheson put forward a new plan whereby all American objectives could be achieved simultaneously. The so-called Acheson Plan sought a 'double *Enosis*' whereby Turkey would be compensated for the unification of Cyprus with Greece. The compensation would be territorial, in the shape of a Turkish military base in Cyprus. Acheson's proposals were as follows:[59]

(1) The full sovereign cession to Turkey, in perpetuity, of a large area of Cyprus for a military base. These areas were located in the Karpass peninsula and the Peristeria-Boghaz region of northeastern Cyprus.
(2) Up to three cantons to be established for the Turkish Cypriots with full local administration in their control.
(3) An international body to observe the application of human rights provisions, with NATO exercising an enforcement role in case of violations.

Acheson later revised some of the provisions in order to secure the agreement of the Greek government. These included the downgrading of the 'perpetuity' proposal to a fifty-year lease to Turkey of a large military base in Cyprus, and delimiting the area of the base to be ceded to Turkey.[60]

Despite its initial agreement, the Greek government had later to reject the plan because of the persistent obduracy of Makarios. A conversation alleged to have taken place between President Johnson and Alexander Matsas, Greek ambassador in Washington, shows the degree of tension which developed between the two governments as a result. When the ambassador told the president that 'no Greek government could accept such a plan', Johnson is said to have replied:

> Fuck your parliament and your constitution. America is an elephant, Cyprus is a flea. Greece is a flea. If these two fellows continue itching the elephant, they may just get whacked by the elephant's trunk, whacked good. [...] If your Prime Minister gives me talk about democracy, parliament and constitution, he, his parliament and his constitution may not last very long.[61]

Notwithstanding these threats, Greece could not accept the plan over Makarios's rejection and a Greco-Turkish war seemed imminent. Knowing that such a confrontation could jeopardise the diplomatic position and possibly the security of the West, President Johnson warned Turkey of the consequences of any unilateral action against Cyprus. In June 1964 he wrote to the Turkish premier that in the event of Soviet intervention against Turkey the United States would not come to its assistance, and thus deterred Turkey from taking any action against Cyprus. Although a costly war between Greece and Turkey may have been averted, the price was high for the United States: its relations with both countries suffered serious strain and intensive work was needed to keep them loyal to the Western camp. By the end of 1964, despite having avoided conflict, United States policy towards Cyprus had failed in two of its objectives: to prevent the internationalisation of the problem, and to contain the communist AKEL. One observer noted in November 1964:

> United States policy-makers appear headed for another setback in the Eastern Mediterranean. The best informed diplomats here agree that Cyprus is likely to hang on indefinitely to its status as a self-governing state. That means the island will probably not become a part of Greece and will not be brought back into the Western Alliance...will be neutralist non-aligned and will play between the Eastern and Western World.[62]

The Soviet Union. Compared with other countries, the role of the Soviet Union in relation to the Cyprus problem was secondary. But one should not underestimate the impact of Soviet policy. it was, after all, the nineteenth-century threat of a Russian advance against the Ottoman empire which led Britain to establish itself in Cyprus and eventually include it among its own colonies. After the Bolshevik Revolution of 1917, communism found its way into the island, and in 1941 AKEL was established. Although communism as an ideology has never appealed to Cypriots, AKEL's support for decolonisation secured the steady support of some 30 per cent of the population.

Soviet policy on Cyprus after the Second World War reflected the bipolarity of the Cold War and Turkey's strategic significance. In the early 1950s Turkey had made strong efforts to join NATO, anxious to escape Soviet pressure for a revision of the 1841 agreement that closed the Bosphorus to non-Turkish warships. Also Turkey wanted to ease Georgian and Armenian territorial demands on its north-eastern borders. It succeeded in joining NATO in 1952: the Soviets then modified their position and sought amicable relations with their NATO neighbour.

The Cyprus issue presented the Soviet Union with two apparently contradictory lines of policy. The first was to take the anti-imperialism stand and support the decolonisation of Cyprus; the second was to alienate Turkey from NATO by taking politically expedient approaches at different times. Any rapprochement between the Soviet Union and Turkey would probably have been detrimental to NATO, and the Cyprus problem offered the Soviets an issue to exploit. By the end of 1964 both of these essentially disparate objectives had been at least partly accomplished.

For the Soviets, *Enosis* was a curious issue. On the one hand, it was a problem because it would automatically take Cyprus into NATO; for this reason AKEL was never a keen supporter of *Enosis* and the Soviet Union was against the partitioning of Cyprus. On the other hand, *Enosis* could prove of value if it could bring about a conflict within the Western alliance. Before the participation of Greece in NATO in 1952, the Soviet Union's policy on Cyprus was a clear case of an anti-imperialist stand.

The London-Zurich Agreements of 1959 provided for a republic from which *Enosis* and partition were excluded. This was a favourable development in the eyes of the Soviet leaders, who also welcomed participation of Cyprus in the Non-Aligned movement. The crisis of 1963 generated the prospect of a NATO peacekeeping force and also a Turkish threat to engage in unilateral action against Cyprus. Neither was in harmony with Soviet policy, because in both cases Cyprus, or at least part of it, would automatically have moved closer to the West. By August 1964 the Soviet Union was indicating clearly that it was ready to come to the assistance of Cyprus in the event of a Turkish invasion. In a statement it declared: 'If a foreign armed intervention takes place in Cyprus the Soviet Union will help Cyprus to defend its freedom and independence...and is willing immediately to start negotiations on this matter.'[63] This warning led to President Johnson's letter already referred to. Towards the end of 1964 Turkey was disillusioned with the NATO membership it had striven for, and saw a rapprochement with the Soviet Union as a possible prerequisite to any desirable development in Cyprus.

Efforts of international organisations at peacemaking in Cypus, 1963-1964

The idea of a NATO force. For all these reasons, the Cyprus crisis caused serious concern in the West. Naturally, there was a keen desire to keep the Soviet Union from obtaining strategic access to the island, and to do nothing which would jeopardise Britain's bases there. Worry was also caused by the threat to NATO arising from the friction between Turkey and Greece over the Cyprus crisis; the alliance's south-eastern flank was particularly exposed and furthermore, the three guarantor powers were all NATO members. Thus Cyprus was 'a state in which the immediate interests of the Atlantic Alliance were involved'.[64] It followed that NATO was viewed – especially by the Union States – as the natural mediator in the Cyprus problem.

In 1958 Paul-Henri Spaak, NATO Secretary-General, tried to involve the organisation for the first time in a peaceful settlement of the dispute, but did not succeed. After the flare-up in 1963, when a war between Turkey and Greece looked imminent, NATO again offered to mediate. The main obstacle now was the Greek-Cypriot leadership – particularly Makarios, who believed that NATO involvement would ultimately undermine the independence of Cyprus. To overcome this problem, the US State Department established contacts with General Grivas, who had directed the military wing of EOKA in the second half of the 1950s and won the admiration of the Greek Cypriots. Through him the United States aimed to gather support among Greek Cypriots for NATO's intervention, despite Makarios's staunch opposition. NATO gained the consent of Greece and Turkey but faced problems later when Makarios managed to persuade Greece to change its mind. The mediation plan itself involved the despatch of a 10,000-man NATO peacekeeping force and the establishment of a NATO base on the island. However, Greek Cypriot objections were expressed by the President of the House of Representatives in Cyprus, who said that it would amount to an occupation by NATO.[65] It was also alleged that NATO's commander-in-chief, (US) General Lemnitzer, had urged the Greek and the Turkish governments to land troops in Cyprus to provide a pretext for NATO intervention, thus presenting the Cyprus government with a fait accompli.[66]

Also entailed in the plan was protection for Turkish Cypriots who chose to remain and compensation for those willing to leave. Meanwhile, the British base in the island would be turned over to Turkey and staffed by Turkish personnel under a Turkish commander.[67]

NATO's plan aimed to achieve a number of important goals. First, it was to contain the crisis and preclude any involvement by the UN. Secondly, it aimed to prevent a conflict between the two parties to the Atlantic Alliance – Greece and Turkey. Thirdly, it sought to block the way to any possible exploitation of the crisis by the Soviets, especially now that Makarios had established friendly relations with them. And finally it was designed to put an end to the Cyprus problem and ensure once and for all a friendly and trustworthy government in Cyprus. To achieve these objectives the power of Makarios had to be curbed. However, backing from the Soviet Union made it all the easier for him to reject the involvement of the Atlantic Alliance. Thus Greek Cypriot objections led to failure of NATO's initiative in 1964.

The question of a role for the United Nations. By 1963 Cyprus was no longer a new issue for the United Nations. From 1954 until the birth of the Cyprus Republic, the UN General Assembly had been presented with the Cyprus problem on four separate occasions,[68] but because of lack of support for the Greek side, no concrete result had been achieved.

The West was deeply concerned over the crisis of 1963-4 and looked for quick measures to re-establish order in Cyprus and avert military confrontation between Greece and Turkey. The Cyprus government was adamantly opposed to any foreign intervention. However, Makarios made it clear in the London conference of 1964 that the UN was the only organisation whose intervention he would accept. On 27 December 1963, the Security Council met to consider a complaint by Cyprus against Turkey over acts of aggression and interference in its internal affairs. On 13 January the UN Secretary-General (U Thant) told the Security Council that the Cyprus government had requested him to appoint a personal representative to look into the situation. Having heard statements by representatives of Cyprus, Turkey and Greece, the Council adjourned.

In 1963 the UN no longer viewed the problem as it had done during the 1950s. By now Cyprus was a UN member with all the resulting advantages: it could ask the UN directly to deal with the problem rather than try to convince Greece to take the issue before it, as had been the case before 1960. Also, Cyprus was entitled as a UN member to ask for help in the protection of its sovereignty, unity and territorial integrity, and for support against any threat. In 1963 the climate in the UN was sympathetic towards Cyprus, since many member states were themselves newly established. It was for these reasons that Makarios preferred the UN to any other intermediary such as NATO. While resorting to the UN was not the first preference of the United States, it was better than the prospect of a Greco-Turkish war, even though it would cost the West some prestige. It also had the advantage of keeping the Soviets quiet, since they had shown interest in the handling of the crisis. Thus in general the UN was the only competent institution to deal with the Cyprus dispute.

In a Report dated 17 January 1964 the Secretary-General informed the Security Council of his decision to designate Lieutenant-General P. S. Gyani of India as his personal representative in Cyprus. Gyani was to observe, for a period up to the end of February 1964, the progress of the guarantor powers' peacekeeping operation in Cyprus, which consisted of military units of the British, Turkish and Greek armies. At the request of the participants in the London conference, on 16 January 1964 the Secretary-General also sent José Rolz-Bennett to London for consultations with the parties concerned. Subsequently on 4 March 1964, as a result of discussions held in and outside the Security Council, Resolution 186 was adopted, setting up a UN peacekeeping force in Cyprus – UNFICYP – for a period of three months and calling for the appointment of a mediator.

The UN force and the proposal for UN mediation. The Cyprus government promptly consented to the establishment of the UN peacekeeping force on the island. As for the force itself, its size and composition were to be determined by the Secretary-General, in consultation with the governments of Cyprus, Greece, Turkey and Britain. The commander of the force would be appointed by the Secretary-General and report to him. The governments providing the force contingents were to be kept informed by the Secretary-General, who was also to report to the Security Council on the operation of the force.

The purpose of UNFICYP was to do its utmost to prevent a recurrence of fighting and contribute to the restoration and maintenance of law and order and a return to normal conditions. The force was to be stationed in the island for a period of three months, and all its costs were to be met by the governments providing the force and by the government of Cyprus itself. The Secretary-General was also authorised to accept voluntary contributions for that purpose.

On 6 March 1964, General Gyani was appointed the commander of UNFICYP. Yet because of political and financial problems with the troop-contributing governments, the force did not come into operation immediately. This was alarming, since Turkey was restive and, only nine days after the adoption of Resolution 186, threatened to intervene unilaterally. On that day – 13 March 1964 – the Security Council adopted Resolution 187, noting the Secretary-General's assurances that the force was about to be established and calling on member states to refrain from actions or threats likely to worsen the situation in Cyprus.

UNFICYP's three-month mandate began on 27 March 1964. Sufficient troops had arrived by then to enable it to fulfil its functions. The

Secretary-General noted that UNFICYP was a United Nations force, operating exclusively under the mandate given to it by the Security Council and, within that mandate, under instructions given by him. It was an impartial, objective body which had no responsibility for political solutions, and would not try to influence events one way or another.[69] The military contingents of the Force came from Austria, Canada, Denmark, Finland, Ireland, Sweden and Britain.

As for mediation, article 7 of the Resolution 186 recommended

> ....that the Secretary-General designate, in agreement with the Government of Cyprus and the Governments of Greece, Turkey and the United Kingdom a mediator who shall use his best endeavours with the representatives of the communities and also with the aforesaid four Governments, for the purpose of promoting a peaceful solution and an agreed settlement of the problem confronting Cyprus, in accordance with the Charter of the United Nations, having in mind the well-being of the people of Cyprus as a whole and the preservation of international peace and security. The mediator shall report periodically to the Secretary-General on his efforts.

It was not an easy choice, since the agreement of all parties was essential if the mediator was to have any chance of success. The task was given to Sakari Tuomioja, who at the time was Finnish ambassador to Sweden and who had a distinguished record. His designation on 25 March 1964 raised no objection from any side. He was briefed in New York and then spent the first two months of his mission in Cyprus.

It should be noted that for the United States the involvement of the United Nations was the last resort. Frustrated with all other avenues of peacemaking in Cyprus – the Acheson and NATO plans – it felt that the UN was the only alternative if the fighting in Cyprus was not to escalate into a Greco-Turkish war. Meanwhile the Soviet Union was gratified to see that, through the Security Council, it had in effect become a party to the Cyprus problem.

As we have seen in this chapter, the crisis of December 1963 was the result of mounting tension and disagreement between the two communities during the first three years of the Republic. The intercommunal tension and mistrust reached new heights at Christmas 1963 as the appeals of the two community leaders for restraint failed to calm the situation.

The Acheson Plan and the NATO Plan were the two distinct peacemaking attempts in the aftermath of the 1963 crisis, but they failed because Makarios was unwilling to grant any foothold to Turkey in Cyprus, or to allow any diminution of his authority. More generally,

Greek Cypriots were against any international peacemaking attempts other than in the context of the UN, and the United States agreed to the UN involvement in the Cyprus problem to stop the escalation of the conflict.

NOTES

1. EOKA: *Ethnike Organosis Kyprion Agoniston* (National Organisation of Cypriot Fighters).
2. Personal interview with Glafkos Clerides, December 1990.
3. See Turhan Feyzioglu, and Necati M. Ertekun, *The Crux of the Cyprus Question*, Lefkosa, 1987, p. 9.
4. Ibid.
5. See Michael Attalides, 'The Turkish Cypriots: Their Relations to the Greek Cypriots in Perspective', in ed. Michael Attalides, *Cyprus Reviewed*, Nicosia, Cyprus: The Jus Cypri Association, 1977, p. 76.
6. AKEL: *Anorthotikon Komma Ergazomenou Laou* (Progressive Party of the Working People).
7. Kyriacos C. Markides, *The Rise and Fall of the Cyprus Republic*, New Haven: Yale University Press, 1977, p. 25.
8. This is a famous statement and is quoted by many. For one source see Dimitri S. Bitsios, *Cyprus the Vulnerable Republic*, Thessaloniki: Institute for Balkan Studies, 1975, p. 23. Also see Hansard, 5th Series, vol. 531, col. 508.
9. Costas P. Kyrris, *History of Cyprus*, Nicosia: Nicocles Publishing House, 1985, p. 314.
10. TMT: *Turk Mughavemat Tashkilat* (Turkish Defence Organisation).
11. See Fazil Küchük, *The Cyprus Question, A Permanent Solution*, Nicosia, Cyprus, 1957.
12. See further, Kyrris, op. cit.
13. Markides, op. cit., p. 25.
14. Ibid., pp 25-6.
15. For further elaboration see Küchük, op. cit.
16. An organisation ('Cyprus is a Turkish Party') set up with the help of Hikmet Bill, a Turkish national.
17. Quoted by Rauf R. Denktash, *The Cyprus Triangle*, Lefkosa, Cyprus: K. Rustem & Bro., 2nd edition, 1988, p. 27.
18. Source does not wish to be identified.
19. Personal interview held with Glafkos Clerides in December 1990.
20. *The Christian Science Monitor*, 6 January 1964.
21. See *The Times*, London 23 October 1961.
22. Glafkos Clerides, *Cyprus: My Deposition*, Nicosia Alithia Publishing, vol. 1, 1989, pp. 175-6.
23. Kyrris, op. cit., p. 380.
24. Ibid.
25. Clerides, op. cit., vol. 1, pp. 149 and 196.
26. Ibid., pp. 149-50.
27. Bitsios, op. cit., p. 116.
28. Thomas Ehrlich, *International Crises and the Role of Law: Cyprus, 1958-1967*, Oxford University Press, 1974, p. 50.

29. W. Miller, 'A New Era in Greece', *Foreign Affairs* vol. 14, no. 4, July 1936, p. 658.
30. Bitsios, op. cit., p. 17.
31. Kyrris, op. cit., p. 364.
32. Stephen Ryan, 'Ethnic Conflict and the International System: Foreign Involvement in the Cyprus Problem, 1974-1982', unpubl. Ph.D. thesis, London School of Economics, 1984, p. 229.
33. Bitsios, op. cit., p. 30.
34. For further details see Adamandia Pollis, 'Intergroup Conflict and British Colonial Policy: The Case of Cyprus', *Comparative Politics* vol. 5, no. 4, July 1973.
35. Quoted by Küchük, op. cit., p. 2.
36. Kyrris, op. cit., p. 368.
37. Harold Nicolson, *Diaries and Letters, 1945-62*, (letter to Juliet Nicolson, 31 July 1954) London: Collins, 1968, p. 311.
38. Kyrris, op. cit., p. 380.
39. See the report by Peter Murtagh, in *The Guardian*, 2 April 1988.
40. Penelope Tremayne, *Below the Tide*, London: Hutchinson, 1958, p. 10.
41. Michael Attalides, *Cyprus: Nationalism and International Politics*, Edinburgh: Q Press, 1979, p. 61.
42. Ibid., p. 9.
43. Ibid.
44. Quoted by Ryan, op. cit., p. 120.
45. George Grivas, *The Memoirs of General Grivas*, transl. and ed. Charles Foley, London: Longmans, 1964, p. 171.
46. Ryan, op. cit., p. 122.
47. Quoted by Ryan, op. cit., p. 122.
48. Markides, op. cit., p. 126.
49. Dundar Aziz, 'The Cyprus Situation', *Pakistan Horizon*, vol. XXVIII, no. 2, 1975, p. 16.
50. Markides, op. cit., p. 129.
51. Bitsios, op. cit., p. 29.
52. Ibid., p. 31.
53. Attalides, 1979, p. 51.
54. Kyrris, op. cit., p. 380.
55. Talk by Rauf Denktash to the Cyprus Sociological Association in March 1974; apparently the only time he has addressed a Greek Cypriot audience.
56. See G. Lewis, *Modern Turkey*, London: Ernest Benn, 1974, p. 203.
57. *Hurriet*, 20 July 1980.
58. See Andreas, J. Jacovides, 'The Cyprus Problem and the United Nations', in ed. Michael Attalides, *Cyprus Reviewed*, op. cit., pp. 200-1.
59. Van Coufoudakis, 'United States Foreign Policy and the Cyprus Question: a Case Study in Cold War Diplomacy', in ed. Michael Attalides, *Cyprus Reviewed*, op. cit., pp. 114-15.
60. Ibid.
61. L. Wittner, *American Intervention in Greece*, quoted by Christopher Hitchens, *Cyprus*, London: Quartet Books, 1984, pp. 61-2.
62. Attalides, 1979, p. 21.
63. Quoted in ibid., p. 141.
64. Quoted in ibid., p. 12.
65. BBC interview with Glafkos Clerides, reported in the *Washington Post*, 31 January 1964.
66. P.N. Vanezis, *Makarios: Pragmatism Versus Idealism*, London: Schuman, 1974, p. 130.

67. E. Weintal and A. Bartlett, *Facing the Brink: An Intimate Study of Crisis Diplomacy*, New York, Charles Scribner's Sons, 1967, p. 33.
68. See Kyrris, op. cit., pp. 364, 367, 368 and 369.
69. *UN Doc.* S/5593/Add. 3, 26 March 1964.

3

THE UNITED NATIONS ATTEMPT AT MEDIATION IN CYPRUS, 1964-1965

Report of the United Nations mediator

In this chapter the Report of Dr Galo Plaza, the UN Mediator for Cyprus in the aftermath of the 1963 crisis, will be outlined and subsequently examined to elucidate the attitudes of the two communities in Cyprus, and of Greece and Turkey. The government of Cyprus, being completely Greek-dominated in the post-1963 era except for some members of the judiciary, continued to be representative of the Greek Cypriot community throughout the period covered by this study.

On 16 September 1964 Plaza was designated by U Thant, the UN Secretary-General, to replace Sakari Tuomioja, who had died suddenly; he was charged with promoting an agreed settlement. Plaza had already acted as the special representative of the Secretary-General in Cyprus and was thus familiar with the problem.

An outline of the Report of the United Nations mediator

Plaza's report was divided into five parts: in parts 1 and 2 he explained his activities and functions in accordance with Resolution 186 of 4 March 1964 of the Security Council; part 3 contained an account of the background to the Cyprus problem; part 4 elaborated on the position of each party involved and the mediation efforts; and part 5 contained the author's observations on the past and the future course of the mediation.

Galo Plaza's recommendations can be summarised as follows:

(1) *Enosis*, since it cannot obtain the agreement of all the parties directly involved, should be excluded from any settlement. This exclusion, however, should not be an imposition on the Greek Cypriots. Rather it should be a voluntary move on the part of the Greek Cypriots in order to bring a peaceful settlement to the Cyprus problem (para. 146).
(2) Cyprus should be demilitarised and refrain from aligning itself with any grouping of nations for military purposes (para. 147).
(3) Partition should be excluded (para. 147).

(4) Federation should be excluded as there is no territorial basis for federation in Cyprus (para. 150).
(5) There should be no return to the pre-1963 conditions in terms of the political partnership of the Turkish Cypriots. The Turkish Cypriots cannot and should not expect the same privileges as those granted to them by the 1960 Agreements (para. 161).
(6) There should be additional and exceptional protection for the rights of the Turkish Cypriots. Those of the Turkish Cypriots wishing to resettle in Turkey should be assisted and compensated (paras 158, 159, 160, 161).
(7) There should be autonomy for the Turkish Cypriots in 'national' traditions, religion, education and personal status (paras 162, 163).
(8) The UN should take the responsibility of being the guarantor of any agreed settlement in Cyprus (para. 168).
(9) The people of Cyprus should either vote for or against any settlement in total and not accept or reject the settlement partially. Any partial acceptance or rejection would disrupt the likely delicate balance of any such settlement (para. 172).

The position of the Greek Cypriots after the 1963 crisis and their attitude to the Report of the UN mediator

Before examining the reactions of the Greek Cypriots it will be helpful to understand the post-1963 situation in Cyprus. After 21 December 1963 Greek nationalism and Turkish nationalism became increasingly a matter of official policy and inspiration in Cyprus.[1] This was not a planned development and took place equally in both communities. The leadership of each began to appear as the embodiment of nationalistic fervour, leading to the polarisation of public attitudes and a propaganda war between the two communities. In his book *The Cyprus Conflict* Zenon Stavrinides writes:

> The Greek and Turkish leaderships needed to arouse and rally their communities around them, and win the sympathy of [the] foreign press and international public opinion. Thus, the Greek and Turkish radio stations, newspapers, politicians and speech-makers plunged into a passionate and vicious propaganda war, attributing evil motives and the worst faith to the opposite side, and especially the opposite side's leaders.[2]

In other words, what up to December 1963 had been a popular movement with the participation of the majority of the Greek Cypriots in the post-1963 crisis, now became an instutionalised instrument in the hands of Greek-Cypriot policy makers in general and of Makarios in particular. This established an authority to be respected by all segments of the Greek-Cypriot community, with Makarios at its head. The separation of the two communities led to the Greek Cypriots taking full control of all the organs of the state, with one or two exceptions. And since this Greek Cypriot-staffed government was internationally recognised as the official government of the Republic of Cyprus, there was little incentive on the part of the Greek Cypriots to try to change the *status quo*, which was that the Turkish Cypriots, who lived mainly in the enclaves, did not constitute a recognisable political entity with the state.

However, there was one serious worry for the Greek Cypriots – the threat posed by Turkey to intervene militarily in accordance with its right under the Treaty of Guarantee. The best way to avoid this, Makarios believed, would be to bring the UN into the problem. Also, on 10 October 1964 the Non-Aligned movement, which Cyprus had been courting, passed a resolution at their conference in Cairo calling for respect for the sovereignty, independence and territorial integrity of the Republic of Cyprus. In terms of gathering international support, then, the Greek Cypriots were rather successful, largely because they were recognised as the legitimate government of Cyprus and enjoyed the sympathy of many newly-established states. 'Unfettered independence' was considered a natural right and any retreat from that position would have been repugnant to the new members of international community.

Added to the international pressure that deterred Turkey was the seeming readiness of the Soviet Union to come to the aid of the government of Cyprus if it were attacked. This in turn led to President Johnson's forceful letter to the Turkish prime minister warning of the grave consequences of any military action against the Greek Cypriots. To all intents and purposes, then, Makarios had achieved a reasonable guarantee against military intervention by Turkey. Greece, of course, promised to defend Cyprus, but this would not have made any decisive impact on its own, since it was no match for Turkey in military terms. Zenon Stavrinides noted:

> It is recognised (though rarely said in public) that Greece is unwilling to go to war with Turkey, because Turkey is militarily not weaker than Greece, and only 40 miles away from the island. A war between Greece and Turkey over Cyprus would result, at the most optimistic estimate, in the territorial partition of the island.[3]

Another consequence of the separation of the two communities was that all financial aid went directly to government of Cyprus[4] and none to the Turkish-Cypriot community. Although some aid did eventually get through, it was after 1965 and not during the crucial period when the UN mediator was preparing his report. In addition, Makarios started an economic blockade, restricting deliveries of food supplies to the Turkish-Cypriot enclaves in Nicosia, Lefka, Limnitis, Kokkina, Famagusta and Larnaca. These restrictions were so severe that towards the middle of 1964, according to some accounts, the population of these enclaves was close to starvation.[5] It was hoped, almost with a degree of certainty, that this economic pressure would eventually cause a crack in the position of the Turkish Cypriots,[6] giving the Greek Cypriots little incentive to reach a quick settlement. Furthermore, in the eyes of the Greek Cypriots the situation after the 1963 crisis had undone the injustices of the 1960 Agreements and there was no need to agree to a settlement that would again compromise their natural rights as a majority.

An important aspect of the 1963 crisis and its aftermath was its military dimension. As the conflict began to spread, the leaders of both communities started to build up their own separate military units as they had done in the last phase of colonial rule. Each party appeared to regard the overall strength of its position in terms of military power: the more armed might it possessed, the more leverage it would have on the course of events and the more concessions it would gain from the other side in any settlement. This arms proliferation, to which Greece and Turkey had also committed themselves, was detrimental to regional and global peace and security. On 17 July 1964 the UN Secretary-General, U Thant, warned the Greek, Turkish and Cyprus governments that their military build-up was increasing the risk of a serious clash. In his book *Burdened with Cyprus*, John Reddaway explains the difficulties then faced by UNFICYP:

> ....The trouble with such peacekeeping forces (and it has happened elsewhere, as well as in Cyprus) is that, as time goes by and there is no settlement of the underlying political problem, their presence tends to freeze the state of affairs as it existed at the time of their intervention, and this may then operate unfairly to the advantage of whichever of the contending parties happened to have the upper hand at the time. As the years go by, a temporary truce thus acquires the character of a permanent settlement. A side-effect is that whichever party gains from a prolongation of the existing state of affairs then has a diminishing incentive to reach a real and lasting solution.[7]

Since in any settlement the military strength of each community would affect the security of the other, the arms build-up continued even after the arrival of UNFICYP and led to military conscription being introduced by the Greek Cypriots in June 1964. General Grivas returned to Cyprus to take over the National Guard.

Another reason for the proliferation of weapons was actual military confrontation between the two communities. Although UNFICYP was generally successful in preventing open hostilities, there were instances when it was unable to do anything. For instance, while it halted the fighting in St Hilarion castle only a fortnight after its arrival, it failed to prevent the Kokkina battle in August 1964 that led to the Turkish air attacks. As a result of their enemy's military superiority, the Turkish Cypriots lost four coastal villages in that battle. Military ability was therefore an essential element if either of the two communities were to gain ground politically or militarily.

As we saw in Chapter 2, Makarios had come to an agreement in 1964 with the new Greek government whereby Greece sent a large number of troops to Cyprus. Their actual number is disputed, with estimates ranging from 3,000 to 20,000, but the likely figure was around 10,000. Makarios also imported arms from Greece and denounced the Treaty of Alliance which allowed Turkey to station troops on the island, on the grounds that the soldiers had refused to go back to their barracks.

The military dimension aside, *Enosis* and Greek Cypriot nationalism remained important issues. There had appeared a separate faction against Makarios which considered him a traitor to the Hellenic cause: a small minority of Greek-Cypriots considered Makarios as an incompetent dictator who clung to power by corrupt means.[8] According to these groups, his charismatic characteristics were Machiavellian traits applied in the service of 'praetorian despotism'.[9]

As the ultimate goal of Greek-Cypriot nationalism, *Enosis* closed doors to other ideas and aspirations which could have been more realistic. Any retreat from it would have been interpreted as a defeat of the Hellenic cause before a minority of Turkish Cypriots. The so-called 'Grivasite' nationalists[10] would not have tolerated any other policy, forcing Makarios, even in reaction to their accusations, to defend the national cause. Neither he nor any other Greek Cypriot official denied the existence of the Akritas Plan, which Turkish Cypriots claim was devised by the Greek-Cypriot leaders to oust them from the Cyprus government before the 1963 crisis – it had been leaked to the Turkish Cypriots.

For the Greek Cypriots the aspiration for *Enosis* had lost its momentum, largely due to the economic prosperity which came to Cyprus after independence. Greek Cypriots, who were more successful in business that their counterparts, started to enjoy a better life in which abstract ideals such as *Enosis* lost their appeal. However, because *Enosis* was the embodiment of national pride they could still be inspired by their leaders to yearn for it.

The points that any mediator would have had to bear in mind on the Cyprus settlement and regarding the Greek Cypriots in the 1964-5 period can be summarised as follows:

(1) Since the leaders of the two communities had become poles in their respective communities, it was important to secure their agreement on any settlement since they would be able to secure the agreement of their respective communities in turn.

(2) Greek Cypriots were in full control of all the organs of the state and had

thus gained from the situation. The problem of Turkish Cypriots would soon be solved, in the Greek Cypriot officials' opinion, through international support for the Greek Cypriots and the economic pressure on the Turkish Cypriots.
(3) Turkey was looking for an excuse to intervene militarily. Any such action would probably drag Greece into the conflict and international peace and security would be at risk.
(4) Greek Cypriots did not accept the 1960 Agreements as a just framework for the structure of the Cyprus government.
(5) Both sides had started a massive build-up of military strength. This was indicative of two important facts: first and foremost it expressed intercommunal mistrust in Cyprus, and secondly it showed that the military strength of each community had an adverse affect on the bargaining position of other community. It should be noted that the Greek Cypriot community had the stronger army in terms of both numbers and armour and ammunition.
(6) Economically the Greek Cypriots were better-off than the Turkish Cypriots. All international aid was going directly to the Greek Cypriots.
(7) *Enosis* was still the official aspiration of the Greek Cypriots although it was gradually losing is appeal.
(8) There was a radical faction which opposed Makarios, believing he had compromised the Hellenic cause. The true attitude of Makarios to *Enosis* is difficult to know for certain: he may have posed as an unwavering supporter of *Enosis* as a reaction to the accusations against him.

The reactions of the Greek Cypriot side to the Plaza Report were mixed: they agreed with almost every recommendation except that which forbade *Enosis*. In a letter to the UN Secretary-General, President Makarios argued that the Cyprus problem 'can only be solved on the basis of the principles of the Charter, as reiterated by the relevant Security Council Resolutions.'[11] This referred to the principle of self-determination by majority.

The position of the Turkish Cypriots after the 1963 crisis and their attitude to the Report of the UN mediator

In 1964 Turkish Cypriots looked to the UN force for 'security and justice,'[12] but they were disappointed. First, Security Council Resolution 186 of 4 March 1964 referred to the government of Cyprus when, according to the Turkish Cypriots, the Greek Cypriots were unconstitutionally and unjustifiably representing themselves as such.[13] According to the Turkish Cypriots this encouraged the Greek Cypriots to continue their unjust behaviour. Also, the UN Secretary-General U Thant is reported to have said that the problem of Cyprus was first and foremost a matter for the Cypriot Government.[14] Referring to the statement in his book *The Cyprus Dispute*, Necati Ertekun comments: 'Such attitudes hardened the Greek Cypriot stand and failed to contribute to an agreed settlement of the Cyprus dispute both then and even now to this day.'[15]

The separation of the two communities has remained a contentious issue ever since the 1963 crisis began. The Turkish Cypriots claim that they were driven out of their homes by the Greek Cypriots and were therefore forced to take refuge in the enclaves. The Greek Cypriots, on the other hand, claim that the Turkish Cypriots imposed isolation on themselves to convince the world that the two could no longer live together in harmony. All the evidence points towards the validity of the Greek Cypriots' claim: an official Turkish Cypriot document leaked to the Greek Cypriots stated that 'a fine of £25 or other severe punishment, and one month imprisonment or whipping' would be imposed on Turks residing in the enclaves who entered Greek areas without special permit, or who did so (permit or no permit) for the purpose of visiting Greek courts, hospitals or other state institutions, or for business with Greeks, or friendly association with Greeks, or merely for a walk or for amusement.[16] In a report to the UN on 11 March 1965 U Thant stated: 'The Turkish Cypriot policy of self-isolation has led the community in the opposite direction from normality.'[17]

A major consequence of the separation was to bring economic suffering. According to some estimates, the Greek Cypriots' blockade on the Turkish Cypriot enclaves and their obtaining all the international aid to Cyprus made as many as one-third of the Turkish Cypriots dependent on relief supplies from Turkey.[18] Indeed from 1964 to 1974 Turkey provided them with an annual income of £10 million.[19] However, it should also be noted that in 1963-4 the value of the confiscated property of the Greeks living in Turkey amounted to £80 million. The dependence of Turkish Cypriots on Turkey increased even further the latter's influence on the policies of the Turkish Cypriot leadership. The basic demand of the Turkish Cypriots was the transformation of the unitary state of Cyprus to a bicommunal one, in which each of the two communities could have its own separate territory. This objective was now partly realised: one effect of the separation was to establish an alternative Turkish-Cypriot quasi-state, with territorial boundaries and a population, which the leadership could effectively control. Their *de facto* administration, however, was not recognised by the international community.

Overall, the points that any mediator would have had to take into account about the Turkish Cypriots in the 1964-5 period can be summarised as follows:

(1) The Turkish Cypriots had imposed a self-isolation upon themselves. They claimed this was for their safety and security. But it may be that they wanted to convince the world that geographical separation of the two communities was the only solution to the problem confronting Cyprus.

(2) They were completely dependent on Turkey for their financial and military needs. Without that help they would not have been able to pursue their policies.

(3) Their policies were very much influenced by Turkey.

(4) Militarily they were inferior to the Greek Cypriots. Their military strength, like that of the Greek Cypriots, affected their political and bargaining position.
(5) They were prepared to engage in bilateral talks with the Greek Cypriots only to restore the 1960 Constitution. Any new solution was to exclude *Enosis*, be bicommunal in nature, and allow for the geographical separation of the two communities.
(6) They had a united front and there was solidarity among the Turkish Cypriots with regard to their bargaining position.
(7) They had a distinct identity in terms of race, religion, culture and traditions. They identified themselves very much with Turkey.

The response of the Turkish-Cypriot leadership to the Plaza Report was negative, believing that the UN mediator had been misled by Greek Cypriot propaganda.[20]

An examination of the UN mediator's Report

It appeared from the position of the two communities that reconciliation was impossible. The Greek Cypriots wanted the rule of the majority – which at the time would have probably led to *Enosis* – whereas the Turkish Cypriots pressed for a bicommunal state. Plaza recorded these positions and recognised that they would have to change if there was to be progress. This was a difficult task for any mediator. Plaza contended that a return to the *status quo ante*, the 1960 Constitution, was unwise, since it had led Cyprus to the 1963 crisis. In paragraph 129 of his report he stated:

> It is enough to observe that the difficulties in implementing the Treaties began almost immediately after independence and became increasingly serious. The events which have taken place in Cyprus since December 1963 have created a situation which makes it psychologically and politically impossible to return to the previous situation. [...] It is obvious that the Cyprus problem cannot any longer be solved by trying to implement fully the Nicosia Treaties and the Constitution governed by the (1960) Treaties.

As such he believed that a new solution to the Cyprus problem had to be found.

Plaza stated that the Cypriot nation had the universally accepted principle of self-determination on its side (para. 143). However, since that would lead to *Enosis* – the biggest problem (para. 136) – it would be opposed by Turkish Cypriots and by Turkey. And since Resolution 186 of 4 March 1964 of the Security Council called for an 'agreed settlement' of the problem, this principle could not be applied (para. 81). But at the same time, the Resolution asked for a settlement compatible with the UN Charter, which in effect supports the principle of self-determination. Here Plaza proposed a way out of the predicament, suggesting that because an individual was limited in the exercise of his freedoms by the welfare of his fellow-citizens, a state in the international community also had to forgo some of its freedoms in the interest of the well being of the whole community (para. 144). As such the government of Cyprus had to bear in mind international peace and security when deciding on its future. Therefore, since *Enosis* could not be agreed to by all the parties concerned, it should be put aside by the free choice of the Greek Cypriots themselves (para. 146). Even if *Enosis* were to be adopted for the settlement of the Cyprus problem, it would bring about many difficulties in terms of integrating the Greek and Greek Cypriot cultures and economies (para. 140), which Galo Plaza had rightly observed to be very different. The Turkish Cypriots' goal of federation (para. 97), meanwhile, was in Plaza's mind an unrealistic solution; his predecessor had come to the same conclusion (para. 81). A federated state would be a constant source of conflict in the island (para. 153), and anyway there was no territorial basis for federation in Cyprus (para. 150). Thus both *Enosis* and federation were excluded from the solution proposed by the UN mediator.

Plaza realised the importance of military power in the position of the two communities. 'Each side rests its widely differing political ideas rigidly, and sometimes menacingly, on the amount of military force at its command' (para. 118). Thus he agreed with Makarios that Cyprus should be demilitarised (para. 147). This would eliminate the fear of armed conflict and the balance between the two sides would not be disturbed by their military strength or weakness.

Perhaps the mediator's most notable failure was to present his report when it was almost certain to be rejected by Turkey and the Turkish Cypriots. There were no signals – at least none were publicly acknowledged – that Turkey would agree with his conclusions and recommendations; on the contrary, there were indications that it would refuse to accept them.[21] It is difficult to assess exactly why Galo Plaza submitted his report when it was unlikely to be accepted by any of the interested parties.

The attitude of the two mother-countries to the Report of the UN meditor

Greece. The Greek government welcomed the Plaza Report – with one notable exception. This was the restraint that he recommended the Greek Cypriots should place on themselves concerning *Enosis*. In a letter to the UN Secretary-General the Greek government said that it

> ....noted with satisfaction that Mr Plaza recognizes the fundamental

> right of people of Cyprus to decide on their own future without any restriction imposed from outside; they are however puzzled that the report recommends self-restraint in the exercise of this right because of the threat of use of force by one of the Members of the United Nations against another Member, since such a threat is absolutely contrary to the provision of the Charter of the United Nations, which the Mediator mentions among the criteria for finding a solution.[22]

Turkey. The Turkish government rejected the Plaza Report on the grounds that he had exceeded his mandate as a mediator and acted as an arbitrator. Its reaction was quick and unequivocal, and in a letter to the UN Secretary-General the Turkish representative at the UN stated:

> The Report of Mr Galo Plaza contains sections which go beyond his terms of reference as specified in the 4 March 1964 Resolution of the Security Council. [...] At any rate, the Turkish Government can no longer expect positive results from the continued mediation efforts of a person who has given vent to his convictions on the substance of the question without the agreement of all parties concerned.[23]

Turkey's outright rejection of the Report put an end to the UN mediation in Cyprus. No progress had been made towards a settlement.

Intercommunal mistrust together with the two communities' different perceptions of a fair solution to the problem of Cyprus were the two main reasons for the failure of Galo Plaza's mediation attempt. The massive military build-up by the two communities and their almost total physical separation were the measure of the mistrust that divided them. Also, while in the Greek Cypriots' view the rule of the majority constituted the premise for a fair solution, Turkish Cypriots thought of federation as a fair basis for a settlement. However, Turkey's unequivocal rejection of the Plaza Report and the qualified Greek support for it indicated the importance of the 'external factors' in the search for a solution. Each community – particularly the Turkish Cypriots – followed the policies of its mother-country towards the report.

NOTES

1. Zenon Stavrinides, *The Cyprus Conflict: National Identity and Statehood*, Nicosia: Loris Stavrinides Press, p. 57.
2. Ibid., pp. 57 and 58.
3. Ibid., p. 65.

4. Ibid., p. 73.
5. Pierre, Oberling, *The Road to Bellapaise: The Turkish Cypriot Exodus to Northern Cyprus*, New York: Boulder, CO: Social Science Monographs, 1982, p. 127.
6. Stavrinides, op. cit., p. 83.
7. John Reddaway, *Burdened with Cyprus: The British Connection*, London: Weidenfeld & Nicolson, 1986, pp. 154 and 155.
8. For a thorough examination of Makarios's power and authority see Kyriascos C. Markides, *The Rise and Fall of the Cyprus Republic*, New Haven: Yale University Press, 1977.
9. Ibid., p. 47.
10. Stavrinides, op. cit., p. 63.
11. Glafkos Clerides, *Cyprus: My Deposition*, Nicosia: Alithia Publishing, vol. 2, 1989, p. 174.
12. Rauf R. Denktash, *The Cyprus Triangle*, Nicosia: K. Rustem & Bro., 2nd edn., 1988, p. 30.
13. Necati Ertekun, *The Cyprus Dispute and the Birth of the Turkish Republic of Northern Cyprus*, Nicosia: K. Rustem & Bro., 1984, p. 19.
14. Ibid.
15. Ibid.
16. Stavrinides, op. cit., p. 58
17. *UN Doc.* S/6228, 11 March 1965, para. 17.
18. Stavrinides, op. cit., p. 81.
19. Ibid., p. 80.
20. Andrew Faulds MP, *Excerpta Cypria For Today*, Nicosia: K. Rustem & Bro., 1988, p. 92.
21. See the official reply of Turkey to Galo Plaza's Report in Clerides, vol. 2, op. cit., p. 164.
22. Clerides, vol. 2, op. cit., p. 173.
23. Ibid., pp. 164 and 165.

4

INTERNATIONAL PEACEMAKING IN CYPRUS, 1965-JULY 1974

An outline survey

The most important event in Cyprus between March 1965, when the Plaza report failed to win the support of the parties concerned, and July 1974, when a Greek-staged coup in Cyprus was followed by the Turkish invasion of the island, was the crisis of November 1967. This underlined once again the importance of peacemaking efforts, drawing the attention of the international community to the explosive potential of the Cyprus conflict and encouraging the process of peacemaking on the island. By 'shuttle diplomacy' the United States once again prevented the conflict escalating into a Greco-Turkish war; and a series of intercommunal talks started under the auspices of the UN. The crisis of November 1967 therefore played an important part in triggering an international response towards peacemaking in Cyprus. Also during this period a military regime took over in Greece, which affected the course of events in Cyprus and subsequently the processes of peacemaking. Ultimately, however, international peacemaking between 1965 and July 1974 failed, although this was perhaps a time when a settlement might have been achieved. During the first two years of this period there was little, if any, activity in the peacemaking front.

The crisis of November 1967

After the rejection of the Galo Plaza report by Turkey and the Turkish Cypriots, a new *status quo* was established. Turkish Cypriots in their enclaves tried their best to live separately from Greek Cypriots. Between December 1963 and the eruption of a new crisis in November 1967 isolated shooting incidents made headlines but did not actually affect the course of events. During this period of uneasy calm, the rhetoric of the two sides continued to boost morale in their respective communities. Typically, a shooting incident would be followed by the mobilisation of forces by Greece and Turkey, requiring the involvement of the UN to ease tension and restore the quasi-normal state of affairs in the country.[1]

In November 1967, however, a serious confrontation which could have led to a Greco-Turkish war occurred in Cyprus around the area of Kophinou. Naturally each side gave a different version of what happened, but the course of events leading to the disaster can reasonably be described as follows. The Turkish Cypriot village of Kophinou is situated on the main road half way between Nicosia and Limassol. Three to four miles to the south lies the mixed village of Ayios Theodoros, and further south is the Turkish Cypriot village of Mari. Despite the existence of a mixed village, the situation in and around these villages was calm. Had it not been for the mixed village of Ayios Theodoros, Turkish Cypriots could have formed an enclave in the area, thus preventing easy passage for the Greek Cypriots between Nicosia and Limassol. Up till July 1967, the Greek Cypriot police used to make regular visits to these villages without any problem, but because of some shooting incidents it had voluntarily abandoned its patrols in the area[2] until it seemed safe and prudent to resume. Later in the year the Greek Cypriot police announced its intention to return, but the Turkish Cypriot fighters claimed that patrolling should not begin until the National Guard had evacuated a recently-created fortification in Larnaca. This rather impertinent reasoning was not well received by the Greek-Cypriot leadership, who interpreted the Turkish Cypriot stand as a step towards ousting the Greek Cypriots from Ayios Theodoros and thus, by creating an enclave, blockading the road from Nicosia to Limassol.[3] The ingredients of a confrontation in the area were therefore all present.

In September the Greek Cypriot police decided to resume regular patrolling in the area, but were turned back by the Turkish Cypriot fighters. Intense negotiations between the Cyprus government and UNFICYP then began to find a satisfactory solution. The Secretary-General himself closely watched developments, and 'when signs of a possible solution had begun to take definite shape, the Cyprus Government felt unable to wait any longer and resumed patrolling from Skarinou into Ayios Theodoros on 14 November, although UNFICYP recommended postponement.'[4] police patrols now moved along the Kophinou-Ayios Theodoros road and entered the village without any resistance; General Grivas, who was commanding an operation code-named 'Feast', spoke to the villagers. The next day, when the Greek Cypriot police moved in they came under fire from the Turkish Cypriot fighters. Having prepared themselves for such an eventuality, the police retaliated with maximum force, and regained control over the villages, but at the cost of some twenty-eight Turkish-Cypriot lives. It was alleged that Grivas went beyond his orders in extending the conflict to the villages and that this was the cause of so many deaths. The Greek Cypriots celebrated their victory, and this exacerbated the situation.

The intercommunal talks, 1968-1974

To give a detailed account of the intercommunal talks between the two communities in the 1968-74 period would require a lengthy and technical scrutiny of the series of the proposals and the counter-proposals exchanged between the two communities in that period, a task for a jurist or student of the constitution of Cyprus.[5] The task here is to present the circumstances in which the talks were held, and the main points which proved crucial to their outcome. There were four phases of talks in the 1968-74 period. The talks in themselves implied a tacit recognition of the Turkish Cypriots by Makarios as a force to be reckoned with; this was a turning point for the Greek Cypriots, since up till then they had seen no need to negotiate with people who denied the legality of the Cyprus government after the 1963 crisis – people whom they called 'rebels'.[6] The crisis in Kophinou and the consequent international pressure for a peaceful settlement led to a change of policy by the Greek Cypriots towards negotiations with Turkish Cypriots.

The first phase (24 June-28 August 1968, Nicosia). The Talks were opened formally on 24 June 1968 at the Ledra Palace Hotel in Nicosia (a preliminary meeting had taken place in Beirut on 3 June 1968). The representatives of the Greek Cypriots and the Turkish Cypriots were Glafkos Clerides and Rauf Denktash respectively. Also present was the special representative of the Secretary-General in Cyprus, Osorio Tafall. From then onwards, it was decided that the two representatives should meet on a regular basis. The talks were to be conducted with an open agenda, each side raising any issue it wished. However, it was agreed to tackle the constitutional issues first and then move on to the question of treaties.[7]

Despite the open agenda, the issue of local government was the topic most discussed between the two parties. No agreement was reached during this phase, but outstanding constitutional issues were identified and it was agreed that further discussion would be held during the next phase of negotiations. The following is part of a statement made by both sides at the end of the first phase:

> This phase covered an exchange of views on the question of the constitutional structure and principles. At this stage we are able to say that there has been identity of views on a number of points and that on others it will not be difficult to establish common ground, but there still remain certain issues, the importance of which cannot be minimised, which require patient negotiations. [...] A break in the talks is needed in order to give us time to make an overall re-appraisal of the views exchange so far and for further consultations with our respective sides.[8]

The second phase (29 August 1968-3 January 1969, Nicosia). In the early meetings of the second phase of the Talks, the Turkish Cypriot side agreed to make a number of concessions if there could be agreement on the question of local government. These included:[9]

(1) The abolition of the vice president's right of veto.
(2) The reduction of Turkish Cypriot participation in the government, House of Representatives, civil service, and the police from 30% to their population ratio (around 20%).
(3) The abolition of the requirement for separate majorities and acceptance of election of the president of the House of Representatives on the basis of a simple majority.

These concessions could only be made, Denktash said, if the powers and functions of local government were clearly defined in the constitution. Makarios, on the other hand, was opposed to idea of local government deriving its powers from the constitution; his aim was 'to reduce the Turkish community's political status to that of a minority, acknowledging autonomy on such matters as religion, education, culture, personal status, but not in local government'.[10] The proposals that the Greek Cypriots submitted on the issue of local government were therefore disappointing to the Turkish Cypriot side; according to Denktash, they did 'not offer a basis for negotiations.'[11]

In a joint statement by both sides at the end of the second phase of Intercommunal Talks, it was stated that proposals on the following points had been exchanged:[12] the judiciary; police; legislation; local government; and the executive. The statement continued: 'We believe that if the present calm atmosphere continues, with patience, understanding and goodwill a just and workable solution can be found.'[13] But the second phase ended without any agreement.

The Third Phase (1969-1970, Nicosia). The main issue during the third phase of the Talks, as in the first two, was local government and the extent to which each side wanted to expand or limit its powers and functions. During this phase the Turkish Cypriot side's views on the question of local government were as follows:[14]

(1) Local government should be based on groups of Turkish Cypriot villages regardless of their geographical cohesion.
(2) There should be separate central government authority for each community.
(3) The powers and functions of local government should be derived from the constitution, and not by delegation of power by the legislature.

The Greek Cypriots rejected all three of these demands. The least contentious issue was the third, on powers and functions.[15]

After it became clear that neither side would make any significant concessions, Denktash agreed to drop his demand on the question of local government, but at the same time he withdrew other concessions he had made on other issues. As he stated to Clerides:

> It seems to me that it might be useful to examine the possibility of finding a solution of the constitutional aspect of the problem without providing a form of local government. [...] You understand, of course, that the Turkish rights I have conceded so far was on the understanding that a satisfactory form of local government acceptable by the Turkish side could be found. Although I accept the principle that some of the Turkish rights contained in the Zurich Agreement should be scaled down, nevertheless I want to make it clear that such scaling down would be to a lesser degree than what my side would have been prepared to concede, had your side accepted the principle of autonomy in local government.[16]

The fourth phase (21 September 1970-July 1974, Nicosia). The fourth phase can be divided into two parts. The first was attended, as before, by the representatives of the two communities and went on for almost a year. The second part, or the 'reactivated intercommunal talks' as they are sometimes referred to, started on 4 July 1972 and ended before July 1974, being attended by representatives from Greece, Turkey and the UN as well as the two communities.

The sticking point was again local government, with the uncompromising stand of the Greek Cypriot side preventing an agreement. In fortnightly meetings during the first part of this phase it became clear that the Turkish Cypriots had made most of the concessions, and that the Greek Cypriot side was not prepared to grant any concessions on the question of local government as wished by the Turkish Cypriots.[17] This stalemate led to pressure on the participants by Greece, Turkey and the UN to include them in the talks, which then reconvened on 4 July 1972. Judge Dekleris, Professor Aldikacti and Osorio Tafall, the Secretary-General's special representative in Cyprus, represented Greece, Turkey and the UN in the talks respectively. However, due to the Greek Cypriots' inflexible stand, these Talks also failed to bring about a settlement, with the sticking point being once again local government. The Turkish Cypriots wanted to retain the autonomy they had acquired in the aftermath of the 1963 crisis but the Greek Cypriots did not want to grant an equal status to the Turkish Cypriots through the provision of local government. Thus the fourth phase failed to produce any agreement between the two sides.

Why the 1968-July 1974 intercommunal talks failed. As a peacemaking mechanism parallel to mediation and accepted by all the parties concerned the intercommunal talks conducted between 1968 and July 1974 in Cyprus were the first of their kind. Although they failed to achieve an agreed settlement, they nonetheless succeeded in identifying the common ground as well as the contentious issues between the two parties. They also brought into the open the concerns behind the policies of the two sides towards each other and clarified the difficulties of reaching a compromise solution. Two main concerns predominated. One was the Greek Cypriots' fear of accepting any agreement that might ultimately lead to partition. This was partly why the most contentious issue proved to be the extent of local government authority and autonomy. These concerns of the Greek Cypriots perhaps were not totally unjustified, as the following quotations from Denktash show. 'Greece and Turkey', he said, 'are the mother-lands of the two communities in Cyprus. In fact Greece and Turkey are in Cyprus through their own communities.' He also considered as 'an unrealistic appraisal of the situation' the view that the 'Cypriots must find a peaceful solution to their problems on the basis of independence without outside interference.'[18]

For its part the Turkish Cypriot leadership suspected that *Enosis* continued to be the ultimate aim of the Greek Cypriots: it was confusing for them to hear one thing from the Greek Cypriot interlocutor assuring them of an independent Cyprus with guarantees for the Turkish Cypriots, and then see Makarios making public statements to the contrary. In an interview on 19 August 1970 Makarios stated: 'I shall never violate my oath, and I shall never deviate from my goal. I have desired *Enosis* and I have never struggled for anything else other than its achievement.'[19] To safeguard themselves against the possibility of *Enosis* becoming a reality the Turkish Cypriots asked for extensive autonomy for local government. The Greek Cypriots, on the other hand, being wary of partitionist desires of the Turkish Cypriots, were unwilling to see government granted such powers. The combination of these two fears on the two sides, which was the direct result of their mutual mistrust, created a situation in which the mistrust on the one side fed and reinforced the same sentiment on the other side. This vicious circle was the main reason for the eventual failure of the talks.

At the beginning of the Talks, positive signs emerged from the Turkish Cypriots when they agreed that the 1960 constitution had been unjust to both communities. They admitted that over-representation and separate municipalities had deprived the Turkish Cypriot community of its young able and educated people in the private sector and placed a heavy financial burden on them.[20] This frank attitude was helpful: another positive element was the fact that the two interlocutors knew each other well from the past. This meant that the atmosphere at the talks was friendly.

The Turkish Cypriots had three basic demands throughout the talks: increased territorially-defined powers for the Turkish Cypriot community, increased autonomy for the Turkish Cypriot community *vis-à-vis* the central organs of the government – or rather an increased tendency to demand that the government of the Republic be composed of the central organs of local government for the two communities – and increased participation by Greece and Turkey in the affairs of Cyprus.[21] During the first phase of the talks, Denktash indicated to Clerides that because of differences of opinion within the Turkish Cypriot leadership he was under urgent pressure to produce some results on the basis of their concessions and their proposals on local government. Clerides recalls:

> The reactions against him of the Turkish Cypriot leadership combined with that of the military together with his inability to solve economic and other problems of his community would, as time went on, lead to a fall in his credibility in the Turkish community, unless he produced results in the intercommunal talks.[22]

At the time Denktash was only the president of the Turkish Cypriot communal chamber, and the leader of the community as a whole was still Küchük. However, when during the last phase of the talks Denktash offered to withdraw the demand on local government and scale down the concessions already made by the Turkish Cypriots, Makarios continued to insist that the concessions remain in place. Clerides observed: 'The view that Turkish community should enjoy only minority privileges and not a partner status continued to be the aim of Makarios to the last.'[23]

A few important developments occurred during this period which in one way or another affected the talks. First, during 1969 political parties were formed by the Greek Cypriots. The initiator of this move was Clerides who founded the Unified Party; other political parties were established soon after. This led to the institutionalisation of the various political approaches prevalent among Greek Cypriots and broke the monopoly of AKEL, which up till then had been the only political party in Cyprus. Although this development in no way undermined Makarios's supreme position among Greek Cypriots, it nonetheless meant that alternative ways to resolve the Cyprus problem could now be aired through the machinery of the political parties.

The second development was the creation of the National Front among Greek Cypriots, which adversely affected the intercommunal talks. This organisation started a violent campaign to eliminate all those whom it saw as obstacles to *Enosis*, including Makarios himself. Despite its illegal activities, Makarios for a while did not outlaw the organisation and contented himself with advising it to dissolve. The Turkish Cypriots saw this development as a possible cause of civil war among the Greek Cypriots,[24] and their confidence in the negotiations was weakened by the inaction of the Greek Cypriots in dealing with the National Front.

A third, very important development during the second phase of the talks was the request by the Turkish Cypriot leadership to those Turkish Cypriots who had left their villages either by force or willingly to return home. This conciliatory move was unfortunately not exploited by the Greek Cypriot leaders, who asserted that certain sensitive areas could not be allowed to be inhabited by the Turkish Cypriots. Thus the first opportunity since December 1963 to resettle the Turkish Cypriots in their own villages where they could be controlled and policed by the government was lost by the Greek Cypriots, and it did not arise again. If they had accepted the offer, the talks in the 1968-July 1974 period might well have benefited. Notwithstanding all the problems, 'a Near Agreement' was reached during 1971-2 which, however, the Council of Ministers of the Cyprus government did not approve.[25] It was the closest the two sides ever got to an overall agreement.

It can be said that the intercommunal talks that started in 1968 showed that gaps could be narrowed – on plenty of the issues, the two communities reached accommodation[26] – but the decisive gap on the issue of local government was the main cause of failure. This difference stemmed from the deep mistrust that prevailed between the two communities, and is why, when towards the end of the talks the Turkish Cypriots appeared to accommodate the Greek Cypriots on the question of local government, withdrawing their other concessions at the same time, the two sides still failed to reach agreement. The 'Near Agreement' of 1971-2 was another manifestation of intercommunal mistrust, for despite its theoretical accommodation of the interests of the two sides, it was not adopted.

The Greek Cypriot attitude to international peacemaking in Cyprus, 1965-July 1974

The Greek Cypriots' attitude to international peacemaking in Cyprus during this period was a mixture of positive and negative elements. Although they agreed to negotiate with the Turkish Cypriots, they nonetheless failed to adopt the positive role needed to settle the conflict peacefully. The objective of the Greek Cypriot leadership throughout the period was to arrive at a solution whereby the Turkish Cypriots were classed as a minority. The crisis of November 1967 was the main factor in persuading the Greek Cypriot leadership to enter negotiations with the Turkish Cypriots, because it had led to the withdrawal of around 10,000 Greek troops from the island and renewed international pressure for peacemaking.

To talk of the Greek Cypriot position is in a sense to talk of Makarios's position. He continued to dominate the affairs of the Greek Cypriots after the Galo Plaza report of 1965, and as president of the Cyprus

Republic he was internationally acknowledged as the leader of a state now completely run by the Greek Cypriots. His victory in the 1968 presidential elections confirmed his dominance of his community: the only candidate to stand against him, a psychiatrist called Takis Evdokas, was heavily defeated – Makarios won a 95.45 per cent majority. This victory was convincing evidence of the support the Archbishop could drum up when he wanted to.

Within the fabric of the Greek Cypriot community, a few changes had come about in the aftermath of the Plaza Report. The most notable was the disenchantment of most Greek Cypriots with the goal of *Enosis*, mainly due to the economic prosperity they had started to enjoy after independence. Their hesitation was reinforced by the military coup of 1967 in Greece – they dreaded the extension of such a dictatorship into their homeland.[27] Among Cypriot officials, however, radical elements who longed for *Enosis* made it difficult for Makarios to distance himself from it publicly. In trying to bring about a balance he played a double act: on the one hand delivering speeches paying lip-service to the goal of *Enosis*, and on the other manoeuvring to stop the Greek government from reaching an agreement with Turkey that would fall short of a complete and total union of the whole of Cyprus with Greece. This balance was difficult to achieve without creating repercussions. Whatever Makarios's true thoughts and intentions on *Enosis*, particularly after the crisis of 1963, he could not accept that the Turkish Cypriot minority should be granted an equal say in the affairs of the state.

In the second half of 1967, the Greek Cypriots were confronted with a problem which proved to be a turning point in the conflict. The period between 1965 and 1967 had been relatively calm partly owing to the presence of the UN force, whose very presence encouraged self-restraint both sides. However, intercommunal tension still existed as the two communities had become entrenched in their positions. The Kophinou disaster in November 1967 brought them to a point of total military confrontation, renewing the risk of a clash between Turkey and Greece. Clerides explained the reasons for the Kophinou disaster as follows:

> Though intercommunal fighting broke out at the end of 1963, the situation in the village of Ayios Theodoros remained calm and police patrols paid it visits at regular intervals. The situation, however, changed in September 1967, when the Turkish Cypriot inhabitants of the village of Ayios Theodoros, encouraged by the commander of about 400 Turkish Cypriot fighters, based in the nearby village of Kophinou, repeatedly prevented the police patrols from entering the village. The object of these actions was obvious.
>
> The Turkish Cypriots, by preventing police access to the village of Ayios Theodoros, intended to cut off the village from the areas

> controlled by the Government, to isolate the Greek Cypriot inhabitants of the village, who having the Turkish Cypriot village of Kophinou, with its four hundred armed fighters on one side, the Turkish fighters of the village of Mari on the other, and Turkish Cypriot fighter groups in their own mixed village, would feel hopelessly outnumbered and surrounded. They would as a result abandon their village seeking safety in the areas controlled by the Government. Thus a new Turkish enclave would be created.[28]

Determined not to give in to the Turkish Cypriots, Makarios and the other members of the Defence Council unanimously decided to take up the issue with the UN. Meanwhile, an important leader of the Turkish Cypriots, Rauf Denktash, was captured by Greek Cypriots off the coast near Famagusta when trying to return to the island from Turkey. However, although a warrant for his arrest and prosecution on a charge of treason had been issued in his absence by the Greek Cypriot authorities, he was released after a preliminary interrogation because, as Clerides writes, there was no admissible evidence against him. Also, his prosecution and conviction would have led to his being widely regarded as a political prisoner, which would have in turn made him 'a hot potato to hold'.[29]

The negotiations between the UN and the two communities failed to provide the Greek Cypriots with the speedy solution to the Kophinou problem they had initially hoped for. Thus as soon as Denktash was freed and left the island, the Defence Council decided to act, resorting to force if necessary, to regain control in the area. It may be that the release of Denktash was linked to this dispute: the Greek Cypriot officials may have feared Turkey's reaction to a simultaneous conviction of Denktash and launching of the Kophinou operation, and set him free to avoid military reprisals. In this case, of course, the Kophinou plan would have had to be agreed before Denktash was freed.

The actual operation in Kophinou began on 14 November, and clashes between the National Guard and the Turkish Cypriots took place on the following day. During the operation the National Guard exceeded its authority in entering the village, which was contrary to the original plan, however necessary it might have been to guarantee military success.[30] Eventually the National Guard succeeded in regaining control over the area and Greek Cypriots celebrated this 'victory' uninhibitedly with maximum press publicity. This was surely a manifestation of immature nationalism, with emotion ruling over political realism. Had the Greek Cypriots kept a low profile over the Kophinou operation the outcome might have been different: as it was, the affair brought serious repercussions for them.

After the crisis Turkey protested in strong terms, and the fear of a Greco-Turkish war once again threatened. As a result of Turkish determination and its overwhelming military superiority, two major concessions had to be made by Greece and the Greek Cypriots: the return to the Greek mainland of General Grivas and of all Greek forces in excess of the numbers allowed by the 1960 Agreements. The latter was of particular significance as some 10,000 troops (the figure varies between 10,000 and 20,000 but the former is generally believed to be more accurate) departed from the island without leaving behind any effective defence force in the event of Turkish military intervention.

In one sense these repercussions favoured Makarios, for as long as Grivas and the National Guard were in Cyprus, he never had as free a hand as he wished: with their departure, he could pursue his own course. And accordingly, on 12 January 1968, he announced for the first time that his policy was to seek a feasible solution, not *Enosis*. On the other hand, the departure of the Greek troops pushed the Greek-Cypriots' morale to its lowest ebb since independence. Also, although the Greek Cypriots still enjoyed military and numerical superiority, the withdrawal weakened their military position and was an important factor in persuading the Greek Cypriot leadership to enter negotiations.

Notwithstanding Makarios's popularity at home, his relations with various Greek governments during this period were, to say the least, uneasy. An example occurred in the summer of 1965, when the Cypriot government, under Makarios, proposed legislation to abolish separate communal voting for the presidency and vice-presidency and membership in the House.[31] The Greek Representative at the UN voiced misgivings about the timing of this move.[32] After the colonels' coup in 1967, Greco-Cypriot relations worsened considerably. Since Athens was known to be '*Ethnikon Kentron*'[33] (the national centre), Makarios's problems with Greece had a serious impact on peacemaking in Cyprus. One of the main consequences of his uneasy relations with the Greek military government was the return of Grivas to the island to take command of all the armed forces of the Cypriot government. Grivas was adamantly opposed to the 1960 Constitution and the Agreements and was a radical *Enosist*. On numerous occasions after his return he acted independently of the Cypriot government, much to the embarrassment its officials.[34] This led to a further loss of confidence in the Greek Cypriots on the part of Turkish Cypriots.

Secondly, the lack of a united front weakened the position of Greece and Greek Cypriots *vis-à-vis* Turkey and Turkish Cypriots and was exploited by Turkey in pursuit of its national interests. Also it brought confusion over the desirability of any particular solution to the Cyprus problem. While Greece wanted a solution within the parameters of its military alliances, specifically NATO, Makarios opposed this as being contrary to Greek Cypriot interests.[35] This discord between Makarios and Greece made the formulation of a satisfactory solution all the more difficult.

An unsuccessful assassination attempt against Makarios in the early 1970s is sometimes attributed to the bad relations between Greece and Makarios. It was later found that the culprits were probably connected to a former interior minister, Polycarpos Yiorkadjis, who was himself shot dead by assassins a week after the attempt on Makarios. Clerides has suggested that the orders to kill Makarios ultimately came from Colonel Ioannides, who arranged the Greek-staged coup against him in 1974.[36] Concerned about the secret return of Grivas to the island. Makarios now started to import weapons from Czechoslovakia to arm his supporters in the event of a Greek plot to unseat him.[37]

Makarios's relations with the Turkish Cypriot leadership between 1965 and July 1974 were minimal. The economic sanctions imposed by Greek Cypriots against Turkish Cypriots remained in place: Makarios calculated that the longer they lasted, the more flexible the attitude of the Turkish Cypriots would become. This might explain the lack of enthusiasm he expressed for the 1968-July 1974 intercommunal talks in a typical statement in August 1969, that 'The margin of optimism regarding that the result of the talks is narrow.'[38] As for the threat of Turkish military intervention, Makarios, like many other Greek-Cypriot officials, was confident that the United States would not allow it.

The Greek-Cypriot approach to the 1968-July 1974 intercommunal talks was naturally dominated by Makarios. For instance, although the Greek-Cypriot negotiator Clerides preferred to be flexible on the issue of local government, he failed to persuade Makarios.[39] The Archbishop's policy towards the talks was confused: his difficult relations with Greece, his fear of an agreement behind his back between Greece and Turkey on Cyprus, the gradual disenchantment of Greek Cypriots with *Enosis*, and the presence of radical Greek Cypriot *Enosists* at high levels in the Cyprus government all contributed to an inconsistent attitude. His determination to treat the Turkish Cypriots as a minority was a major cause of failure: it seemed unfair to him, as perhaps also to others in the Greek-Cypriot establishment, that a mere fifth of the population should be granted the status of a partner.[40] Had it not been for this the talks might have succeeded. In the words of Clerides, '....1964 to the end of 1970 was a period during which the Cyprus problem could have been solved.'[41]

The Turkish Cypriot attitude to international peacemaking in Cyprus, 1965-July 1974

The 1965-July 1974 era was the period when the Turkish Cypriots became a force to be reckoned with and their leadership entered into negotiations with Greek Cypriots. They managed to stay separate from

Greek Cypriots and run their affairs independently, but suffered as a result from a poor economy and a low standard of living.

The Galo Plaza Report, in their view showed ignorance of their needs and problems. They now argued that the 1963 crisis had proved once and for all that the two communities could not live together in harmony,[42] and that the Greek Cypriots clearly aimed at Enosis as the ultimate goal of the Cyprus Republic. Rejecting Greek Cypriot allegations that labelled them as insurgents trying to sabotage the state, they pointed out that if the 1960 Agreements had been so favourable to their community, they would have had no reason to abandon them.[43] Far from seeking isolation, they insisted, they had been driven into enclaves. To prove this, they were eager to point out that their representatives were prevented from entering the House of Representatives in July 1965 'unless the Turkish deputies agreed to the abrogation of the constitution and endorsed the unconstitutional laws enacted in their absence by their Greek counterparts.'[44] In this connection Kyriakides also writes:

> The Greek Cypriot leadership believes that the Turkish Cypriots have abandoned the government in order to undertake a rebellion against the Republic. To the Greeks, therefore, all actions and laws enacted by the government, without the consent of the Turkish Cypriots, are binding. If the Turkish Cypriots wish to 'return' and cooperate with the government, they must first accept the legality of the laws enacted during their 'absence'.[45]

However, as we have seen, the Turkish Cypriot isolation seems on the whole to have been imposed on the community leadership. Maintaining a separate administration was by no means easy since it was subject to an economic embargo which, without help from Turkey, would certainly have forced the Turkish Cypriot leaders to compromise with the Greek Cypriots. In fact the Turkish Cypriot economy was so stagnant that, according to UN estimates in December 1966, approximately one-third of the people needed some sort of relief.[46] They also suffered psychological pressure – what the UN Secretary-General U Thant described as 'too many cases of close bodily searches and lengthy interrogations which [did] not appear to be justified by the need to look for arms and strategic materials'.[47] Furthermore, the prolongation of the dispute was seen by Turkish Cypriots as a source of prosperity for the Greek Cypriots.[48] The validity of this claim would be for economic historians to decide, but on the surface it does not seem justified. A more accurate description of the economic situation might be that the effect of prolonging the dispute was to worsen poverty in the Turkish Cypriot areas rather than create Greek Cypriot prosperity, which is why Makarios thought that time was on the side of the Greek Cypriots.

In the period following the Plaza Report, the Turkish Cypriot leadership managed to assert effective control of its population, but not in a well defined and cohesive territory. Politically it had an administration, but no legal state existed apart from the internationally-recognised state of Cyprus. Stavrinides writes on the Turkish-Cypriot administration:

> ...although it lacked the name of a state, what the Turkish Cypriots created was in essence a small national state, existing within defended borders, with its own government (called after December 1967 the Turkish Cypriot Administration), public services and even luxuries like a Football Federation and a Scouting Movement.[49]

But the core of the problem for Turkish Cypriots remained the Greek Cypriots' determination to merge with Greece,[50] as this public statement made by Makarios on 26 May 1965 seemed to confirm:

> 'Either the whole of Cyprus is to be united with Greece or [it will] become a holocaust. [...] The road to the fulfilment of national aspirations may be full of difficulties, but we shall reach the goal – which is *Enosis* – alive or dead.'[51]

The Kophinou crisis was, in the Turkish Cypriots' view another manifestation of their enemy's determination to annihilate any resistance to *Enosis*. After the incident and the withdrawal of Grivas and the Greek troops from the island, the Turkish Cypriots learned that Turkey was a reliable supporter and that Greece could not afford to go to war with her, which greatly boosted their morale and emboldened them to declare a 'Temporary Separate Turkish Administration' in the areas under their control.

From this new position of strength, the Turkish Cypriot leaders entered the intercommunal talks demanding autonomous local government. However, although they seemed willing to accommodate the objections of the Greek Cypriot side on local government, it is difficult to ascertain whether they wanted a final agreement. First, because the Turkish Cypriots depended on Turkey for their survival, they could not agree to a solution without Turkish consent, and it also cannot be established that at the time Turkey unreservedly wanted a solution of the Cyprus problem. Secondly, the Turkish Cypriot mistrust of Greek Cypriots over *Enosis* was paramount, and without extensive local government autonomy, this fear would probably have counterbalanced any advantage from a settlement.

Overall, the Turkish Cypriots' attitude to the international peace initiatives was widely believed to be influenced by the Turkish government. However, their willingness to go the extra mile by agreeing to withdraw their demands on local government made their position more positive than that of the Greek Cypriots.

Outside powers and international peacemaking in Cyprus 1965-July 1974

The United Kingdom. Britain's policy towards peacemaking in Cyprus between 1965 and July 1974 was one of inaction; there was no British initiative. After the failure of the London conference in 1964 to bring about an agreement between the parties, George Ball, President Johnson's appointee to deal with the Cyprus problem, came up with a plan to establish a joint peacekeeping force consisting of Britain, Greece and Turkey to patrol the island. When Britain rejected the plan, Ball complained that it wanted to a divest itself of any responsibility for Cyprus.[52]

However Britain's position over UNFICYP was already important since it could offer invaluable help through its military bases on the island. It also provided the largest contingent of troops. The deputy commander of the force was at first General Young, later replaced by General Carver. Britain's interests after relinquishing sovereignty over Cyprus remained the same: to safeguard its sovereign bases and the intelligence headquarters in the Troodos mountains, but its military presence also helped to defuse tension between the two communities. In 1967 the Defence and Overseas Policy Committee of the British Cabinet discussed a Cabinet paper that proposed to condemn, but not use force to prevent, any attempt by the Greek military regime to stage a coup in Cyprus and proclaim *Enosis*. Richard Crossman and Denis Healey were strongly critical of the proposal, calling it, in Crossman's words: 'totally intolerable', and the passage was deleted.[53] In a *Guardian* article of 1988, Peter Murtagh suggested that the British government in the 1960s preferred to divide rather than re-integrate the two communities and described the case of British officers who, despite or perhaps because of successful initiatives in bringing the two communities together, were recalled from the island and had their reports supressed.[54] It is of course no secret that the ideal US solution to the problem was that proposed by Dean Acheson – namely partition. It is also true that Britain and the United States followed the same or parallel lines of foreign policy in many parts of the world. However, the allegation that Britain deliberately aimed to divide the two communities in Cyprus cannot be substantiated. A more obvious reason for British inaction may have been its unwillingness to bear responsibility for any failure, particularly after the problem of Northern Ireland erupted in 1969. It was reluctant to get involved in another conflict where intercommunal strife was the source of the conflict.

One important development over the sovereign military base of Dhekelia should be noted. Between 21 March 1966 and 17 December 1966, the Stefanopoulos government in Greece made many efforts to find out whether the British government would be willing to cede

Dhekelia base to Turkey if an agreement could be found between Greece and Turkey over Cyprus. Extensive talks had been held on the subject of the base between the two mother-countries. Clerides describes the British government's reply as follows:

> In the event Greece and Turkey could reach an agreement on the Cyprus problem, which would have also the agreement of the government of the Republic of Cyprus and of the Turkish Cypriots, then the British government would examine with sympathy any common proposal of the interested parties regarding the future of the British Base of Dhekelia.[55]

After the formation of the National Front among Greek Cypriots, the British high commissioner, Mr Ramsbotham, expressed his anxieties over the group's activities.[56] He also stated his pessimism over the intercommunal talks and proposed that economic cooperation should seriously be considered until an agreement was reached.[57] In sum, the view that a wish to maintain the *status quo* between 1965 and July 1974 was the reason for British inaction would seem unjustified: only a year earlier, in 1965, Britain invited all the parties to London with the express purpose of seeking a solution. What is more likely is that Britain was fully aware of the irreconcilable positions on both sides and was not keen to engage in futile negotiations. Nor did it want to upset the Muslim world by pressurising Turkey into a settlement, even assuming it was in a position to do so.

Greece. Greece's attitude towards peacemaking in Cyprus in the 1965-July 1974 period was rather confused, mainly due to the rapid succession of governments and the inexperience and crudeness of the military regime that took power in April 1967. The dictatorship was intent on bringing an end to the Cyprus problem, but was never clear how this was to be achieved. Greece's contribution to peacemaking efforts in Cyprus over the 1965-July 1974 period must be considered to have been negative.

To begin with, relations between Greece and Cyprus during and before the 1968-July 1974 talks were not easy. Their differences following the independence of Cyprus can be traced back to 1963, when Makarios ignored the strong advice of the Greek premier, Karamanlis, against introducing thirteen amendments to the constitution.[58] The caretaker government of Paraskevopoulos advised Makarios to accept the Acheson Plan for stationing a NATO force and a NATO mediator in Cyprus. Makarios rejected this also, as he did George Papandreou's later recommendation of the second Acheson Plan. Papandreou also warned the Archbishop against using military force which he feared could lead to a Greco-Turkish war, but Makarios was prepared to use force if necessary. In their turn the military rulers of Greece were aware that at the end of 1966 the previous government had been accused openly by the Cypriots of having spies in the National Guard of Cyprus and of mishandling the Cyprus problem.[59] An assassination attempt against Papadopoulos, the head of the Greek military regime (1967-74), was later linked to the Greek Cypriot minister of the interior, who was forced by Greek pressure to resign,[60] further damaging relations.[61] These disagreements seriously undermined international peacemaking efforts in Cyprus and weakened the Greek/Greek Cypriot front *vis-à-vis* the Turkish/Turkish Cypriot front in negotiations.

A major turning point in Greek politics with serious consequences for Cyprus occurred on 21 April 1967 with the coup that led to the establishment of a military government in Athens. Greco-Cypriot relations were a two-way street: although Greece as the mother-land was publicly acknowledged as the 'National Centre' and thus a major shaper of Greek Cypriot policy, Cyprus also affected Greek politics through the position of Makarios as Ethnarch and the fact that the problem of Cyprus could arouse emotions on the mainland – so much so that, according to the *Guardian*, one of the main reasons for the military take-over in Greece was to solve the Cyprus problem one way or another.[62]

The military regime saw itself as the saviour of Greece from instability and anarchy. Domestically it provided stability through repression. Over Cyprus the national aspiration was still, officially at least, for *Enosis*; in fact two years before the coup, in May 1965 (in Athens), Makarios had proposed that *Enosis* be proclaimed if the Greek government of the time would support him. In response the prime minister George Papandreou had prevaricated, arguing a price would have to be paid to Turkey and if this turned out to be too high, constitutional changes in an independent Cyprus should take priority instead.[63] Lacking popular support at home and in the face of widespread criticism abroad,[64] the military rulers relied heavily on American support; indeed this dominated their policy on Cyprus. After Papandreou governments had used the Greek military in Cyprus as an instrument of policy, leading to subversion and the formation in 1969 of the National Front, which according to a report in *Der Spiegel* sought 'double *Enosis*', or partition. The junta's basic aim was more or less what the US Secretary of state Dean Acheson had proposed a few years earlier – *Enosis* in exchange for territorial concessions to Turkey.

To try to get an agreement with Turkey the Greek military regime sought a dialogue, but talks in September 1967 at Kesan-Alexandropolis ended in failure because of the Greek insistence on *Enosis*.[66] So struck were the Turks by the inexperience of the Greek negotiators that the Turkish foreign minister described it as the biggest farce he had ever witnessed.[67] Two years later the Greek government resumed its contacts, culminating in June 1971, at a NATO conference of foreign ministers, with an agreement over terms to divide the island.[68] Earlier the dictatorship had been preparing the ground for cooperation with Turkey. Papadopoulos, head of the military junta, said in an interview on 30 May 1971 that the two countries: 'should convince our communities in Cyprus that we are not disposed to spoil the relations between us and quarrel for their sake; consequently they should settle their differences in a manner acceptable to us.'[69]

Besides winning favour with the United States, the Greek Colonels had other reasons for undermining the independence of Cyprus. A democratic Cyprus with a charismatic ethnarch as its president was a menace to the repressive Greek regime. Secondly, Makarios had appeared to support the growth of communism on the island: his links with AKEL and his importing of weapons from Czechoslovakia to arm his supporters against EOKA-B (the organisation formed and commanded by Grivas in the early 1970s and aimed at bringing about *Enosis*) reinforced this belief in Greece. The Colonels acted strongly over the importation of the arms, and insisted to Makarios that they be handed over to UNFICYP at once.[70]

While the idea of an independent Cyprus, with all that this entailed, was unsettling to the Greek military regime, the way the Greek junta conducted its policies towards Cyprus suggests a dichotomy of objectives. At the same time as trying to strike a deal with Turkey over the division of Cyprus, it was pressing the Cyprus government to remedy the slowness of the 1968-July 1974 intercommunal talks by granting concessions on the question of local government. The Greek foreign minister, Pipinelis, is quoted as telling the Greek Cypriots that his government believed that the 'intercommunal discussions were the most appropriate procedure for arriving at a mutually satisfactory internal constitutional settlement.'[71] This contradiction can be attributed to either of the following theories. One is that within the Greek junta there were still those whose military zeal did not outweigh their political realism. Despite the military trend of the time, these people were more lenient towards the Greek Cypriots in preferring a solution that had the agreement of Makarios. A second theory suggests that Greek policy wanted the intercommunal talks to result in local autonomy for the Turkish Cypriots, thus opening the way for partition. The dual policy of Greece was conspicuously noted by Makarios in the following statement:

> The Greeks were being two faced. On the diplomatic side, they were stressing independence for Cyprus while on the military side the officers shouted every day for Enosis. Always the Greek military were trying to undermine the intercommunal talks.[72]

The Archbishop went on a visit to Greece in 1971, his last during the reign of the junta. During this visit he was asked to accept the agreement reached at a NATO conference in Lisbon between Greece and Turkey. Makarios reportedly objected and refused to abide by the agreement.[73] In the same year the Greek military dictator put to the US government the idea of removing the Archbishop through a coup if he failed to respond positively to pressure.[74]

The Greek military regime was highly autocratic, not least over peacemaking in Cyprus: it sent King Constantine into exile following his failed attempt to oust it in the aftermath of the Kophinou disaster. The following remark concerning Cypriot politics by General Grivas demonstrates their mentality: 'Give me a whip...and I will show you what I can do. What are these things? Parties, para-parties, conflicting factions and para state organisations. Let them give me a whip and then we can talk again.'[75]

All this suggests that after the coup of 1967, the main problem for Greece became Makarios rather than Turkey. This had a serious negative impact upon peacemaking in Cyprus since Greece was thought to have the most influence with Greek Cypriots. Yet diplomatically the regime was unable to outmanoeuvre the Greek-Cypriot President and militarily its influence was reduced after its troops were evacuated from the island after the Kophinou operation. With hostility at home and abroad and jockeying in the military ranks for leadership, the regime found itself being ignored by the Greek Cypriots. For Greece, the 1965-July 1974 period was a gloomy one where peacemaking in Cyprus was concerned.

Turkey. Turkey's impact upon peacemaking in Cyprus in the 1965-July 1974 period was significant. As the sole supporter of the Turkish Cypriots and their administration, it was in a strong position to steer the course of policy pursued by their leadership, and as a guarantor power, like Britain and Greece, it closely followed the course of events on the island. Its main concerns continued to be security on its southern coast and anxiety over the wellbeing of the Turkish Cypriots. The strategic importance of Cyprus for Turkey can hardly be overstated, and far exceeds its strategic significance for Greece.[76] As such, its fears centred mainly on *Enosis*, especially after President Johnson's warning letter in 1964, which together with Soviet support for Makarios, ruled out the use of military force. Obligations to NATO also restricted its choice of action.

The crisis of 1963-4 had created indignation in Turkey. Despite public pressure and an authorisation given on 16 March 1964 by the parliament to the prime minister, Inönü, to use troops against the Greek Cypriots,[77] the government was unable to comply. However, after the formation of Turkish Cypriot enclaves, it dispatched an officer to each one to coordinate military matters. According to Michael Harbottle it was one of these Turkish military advisers in Ayios Theodoros, Mehmet, who was the primary cause of all that was to follow.[78]

Domestically Turkey was under pressure to act in support of Turkish Cypriots and against Greek Cypriots. It was already committed to Cyprus financially, undertaking the expensive task of providing aid to the Turkish Cypriots during the economic blockade, which according to some estimates amounted by 1966 to an equivalent of £8 million anually.[79] However, Turkey's problem was not the financial burden but rather, as some have suggested, the lack of strong and decisive government action in Ankara. In October 1965, however, the period of weak coalition governments came to an end as the Justice Party won the majority of seats in the National Assembly. Oberling has described the change of government:

> The new premier, Suleyman Demirel, was determined to act decisively if provoked by some blatant act of aggression against the Turkish Cypriots, and he was under growing pressure to adopt a firm policy towards the Makarios regime from the Turkish population which favoured a military solution to the Cyprus problem.[80]

Internationally, Turkey enjoyed a better climate where its policies over Cyprus were concerned after the publication of the Galo Plaza Report. Its strategic position was particularly important to the balance of power in the eastern Mediterranean between the two superpowers. Wooing Turkey had been a Soviet objective for some time:[81] in the late 1960s a series of top-level official visits led to closer ties and an eventual shift of Soviet policy, to the extent that Moscow now criticised Czechoslovakia for continuing to export arms to Cyprus. Aware also of the United States' disenchantment with Makarios, Turkey felt more confident about that superpower's Cyprus policy.

The Kophinou disaster was in a way a test case for the new government in Turkey, leading to pressure from the military and public opinion which, unlike the situation in 1963, could not be ignored. The official reaction to the incident appeared in a statement issued by the Turkish foreign minister:

> The attack launched against the Ayios Theodoros area has introduced an element of complication such as had not been seen since 1964. Such action, while there was still a possibility of reaching a negotiated solution of the Ayios Theodoros problem (meaning patrolling by the Cyprus police), constitutes a flagrant provocation by the Cyprus government. UNFICYP is requested to stop the fighting immediately and clear the Turkish Cypriot areas of Ayios Theodoros and Kophinou of both Greek Cypriot and Greek armed forces. If this cannot be done, a crisis which will go beyond the borders of the island will be unavoidable.[82]

Following the ceasefire, the Turkish government demanded the following:[83]

(1) removal of all Greek troops from Cyprus in excess of those allowed under the treaties;
(2) immediate withdrawal of General Grivas;
(3) compensation for the Turkish Cypriot victims of the recent attack;
(4) relaxation of all restrictions on the Turkish Cypriots;
(5) effective guarantees against any further attacks on the Turkish Cypriots;
(6) enlargement of the United Nations peacekeeping force to prevent further attacks; and,
(7) disbandment of the National Guard.

Some of these demands, such as the withdrawal of General Grivas and of Greek troops, were met, but others, notably the enlargement of UNFICYP, were not. In advancing these requests Turkey took two main considerations into account. First the junta in Athens was in a vulnerable position internationally, which could only be worsened by a confrontation with Turkey. At the same time the Colonels were unlikely to be displaced in the near future, so any agreement might last for a considerable time. Added to this was the growing disenchantment of the Greek military regime with Makarios, which meant that he would not be able to veto any agreement struck between the two mother-countries. The second consideration was the reaction of the two super-powers to its demand, which it put forward as much as anything to test their reactions. The result was satisfactory: this time no warnings were issued by the US president against Turkish military intervention, nor did the Soviet Union threaten to come to the aid of Cyprus in such an eventuality. This emboldened Turkey in its attitude to Cyprus.

The initiative for the talks apparently came from Turkey.[84] The position of the Turkish government towards them has been summarised by Necatigil as follows: the intercommunal talks should be encouraged; both *Enosis* and partition should be excluded; the difficulty of the problem should not be underestimated; and the discussions were bound to be long and arduous, but they might be the last chance for peace.[85] Turkey's aims during the talks, as understood by the then Greek foreign minister, were the preservation of the unitary state of Cyprus and identity of the Turkish Cypriot community.[86] Turkey complained to Greece of the slow pace of the Talks; with elections coming up in 1969, it was willing to take steps to facilitate a speedy resolution and this consideration may have been why it initiated the return of Turkish Cypriot refugees to their homes – a positive move of which Makarios failed to take advantage. Another Turkish proposal was a five-party conference consisting of the three guarantor powers, the Cyprus government and the Turkish Cypriots' representatives. The idea was opposed by Greece, but it put pressure on them and the Greek Cypriots to be more positive in their attitude towards the intercommunal talks. Then the 'coup by memorandum' of 1971 brought the Demirel government down and caused a temporary interruption of the talks. The new premier, Erim, took a harder line on Cyprus.

Turkey's impact on peacemaking in Cyprus in the 1965-July 1974 period was most significant since it was the sole financier and supporter of Turkish Cypriots. It exerted its influence among Turkish Cypriots for a settlement, and tried to come an agreement with Greece. Although it is difficult to establish unequivocally that Turkey genuinely wanted a settlement, it can be argued on the basis of available evidence that it favoured one, partly because of the dramatic improvement in its relations with Greece, its NATO ally, that would follow. As the Turkish foreign minister said in 1969, 'There is no doubt that the Cyprus question is the foremost factor in our relations with Greece.'[87]

The United States. In the 1965-July 1974 period the Cyprus conflict was taken seriously in the United States because of its potential to drag Greece and Turkey into war. However, the United States and Makarios disagreed over how a solution was to be brought about.

Following the publication of the Plaza report, US policy towards Cyprus was shaped by its Cold War diplomacy. The Acheson Plan expressed the containment policy of the State Department and its failure to secure the agreement either of Makarios or Greece meant another solution had to be found. The United States had already tried through NATO to send a peacekeeping force to the island, but this too had been vetoed by Makarios. In the meantime, its proposal for a summit of the heads of the guarantor powers was rejected by Britain.[88]

To achieve the all-important objective of averting a Greco-Turkish war, a new method had to be adopted. Other objectives included a ban on AKEL and the continued inclusion of Cyprus within the Western camp. The latter became more important in the light of certain regional developments: the six-day Middle East war of 1967; the prospect of a re-opened Suez Canal; the loss of American base rights in Libya; and the improved position of the Soviet Union *vis-à-vis* some Arab states.

After the crisis of 1963-4 the most immediate concern of the United States was to prevent any escalation of intercommunal fighting in Cyprus. Although President Johnson's June 1964 letter had averted a war between the two NATO allies, there was no guarantee that this would succeed a second time. United States relations with both mother-countries, particularly Turkey, had already been adversely affected; Cyprus was a potential source of friction between Turkey and Greece, a constant embarrassment to the Western alliance and an important factor in superpower rivalry.

UN involvement was not necessarily an adverse development for the US administration, because although it eased Soviet concern by making the use of force less justifiable, it also helped to lower tension between Greece and Turkey. It therefore received considerable US and NATO support.[89] However, this marriage of interests did not last long. Twice in 1965 differences surfaced between the United States and the UN. The first occasion was when the Galo Plaza report was issued, calling for a solution from within in the context of the unitary state of Cyprus, as against the US preference for settlement along the lines of the Acheson Plan, which required the dissolution of the Cypriot state. And when on 18 December 1965, at the request of the Cypriot government, the General Assembly adopted Resolution 2077 (XX) calling on all states to respect the independence, sovereignty, unity and territorial integrity of the Republic of Cyprus,[90] only a handful of countries supported the United States in voting against it.

At the centre of US disenchantment with the Cyprus problem was Makarios. It was he who had rejected the NATO force option, and who had rejected the Acheson Plan and persuaded the Greek government to do likewise. AKEL was operating with the Cyprus government, with support and encouragement from Makarios. He had also joined the Non-Aligned movement and internationalised the problem by repeated recourse to the UN. Ultimately, American policy-makers regarded Makarios as a threat to regional security and an obstacle to the achievement of American objectives. George Ball expostulated: 'That son of a bitch Makarios will have to be killed before anything happens in Cyprus.'[91]

The tension with Makarios strengthened the belief of the United States that Greece was best placed to bring the Cypriot president into line with US objectives, and this has been viewed as the main factor behind the American-sponsored ousting of George Papandreou in 1965.[92] According to a US Congressional mission:

> The United States, despite an official policy of neutrality and non-intervention in Greece's domestic affairs, appears to have sided, throughout 1965-67, with King Constantine (and the conservative forces which had coalesced around him) and against George Papandreou. Apparently the conservatives were expected to take a more moderate (i.e. pro-NATO) line *vis-à-vis* Turkey on the subject of Cyprus.[93]

Having failed to bring about a favourable solution directly, the State Department decided to implement its policies in Cyprus through Greece and Turkey. This rather more realistic approach was mainly a result of frustration with Makarios, whose skilful diplomatic manoeuvring at the UN and elsewhere had practically outwitted the Americans. Moreover, direct American action would have provoked a new Soviet propaganda campaign and pressure for concessions elsewhere. Also, any solution reached by the two mother-countries would probably enjoy the support of their respective communities in Cyprus, which would make it appear more legitimate than any US plan such as Acheson's.

The seizure of power by the Colonels in 1967 was condemned in most of the world. Nevertheless, the US administration, in spite of expressing reservations, was not actually opposed to the military government – on a visit to Greece, Vice-President Spiro Agnew and US admirals leaped praise on the Colonels.[94] The new rulers' anti-Communist stand and their keenness to keep the American bases in Greece were good reasons for US support.

The crisis of 1967 again raised the possibility of a Greco-Turkish war. In view of the rapprochement between the Soviet Union and Turkey, any attempt by the United States to deter Turkey from entering a war with Greece carried a risk of pushing Turkey into the arms of the Soviets. At this point, on 22 November 1967, President Johnson sent Cyrus Vance, a former Deputy Secretary of Defence, as his Special Envoy and by means of what would later be called 'shuttle diplomacy' – constant travelling between the three capitals, Athens, Ankara and Nicosia – Vance managed to reach a compromise. As we have seen, this was facilitated by concessions mainly from Greece, made under pressure from Vance.[95] However, the Greek agreement to withdraw troops indirectly helped to strength the independence of Cyprus and reinforce the position of Makarios. Since, as we saw, their presence on the island limited his freedom of action in the context of worsening relations between Greece and Cyprus. By pressurising Greece to withdraw its troops from Cyprus, the United States thus eliminated the only effective obstacle to Makarios and emphasised the importance of averting a war between Greece and Turkey.

The intercommunal talks enjoyed American support for three reasons: Makarios's skilful diplomacy, the enhanced strategic importance of Cyprus following the 1967 Arab-Israel war, and the Soviets' diplomatic presence which made the imposition of any solution from the West very risky. A peaceful solution through dialogue between the two communities seemed preferable to Americans, unless contacts between the two mother-countries could lead to an agreement between them, in which case the talks could merely ratify it. American policy-makers, though aware of the impracticality of the Acheson Plan, still favoured the kind of 'two-community' solution openly supported by President Johnson during a visit to the United States by the then Turkish President, Sunnay, in April 1967.[96] This would have limited Makarios's influence, as the Turkish Cypriots did not have an organised left corresponding to AKEL in the Greek Cypriot community.

The authority of Makarios was weakened by the return of General

Grivas to Cyprus in the early 1970s. Besides this, Grivas might be able to persuade the Greek Cypriots to drop their objections or the local government issue in the intercommunal talks. Grivas and his National Guard were regarded by the American ambassador in Nicosia, Poper, as the 'joker in the pack',[97] which could be used in any future development.

By early 1973, US officals decided to press for a reduction in the number of soldiers in UNFICYP, for two reasons:[98] the mounting cost of maintaining the force[99] and the fact that the *status quo* that UNFICYP tended to maintain worked, in their view, to Makarios's advantage. US influence in Cyprus in the 1965-July 1974 period has been exaggerated but at the same time it should not be underestimated. The Greek Colonels believed that about 90 per cent of any solution would have to come from the Americans,[100] which is perhaps something of an overstatement. On the other hand, the importance of Cyprus to Washington cannot be taken lightly. In the words of a West German strategist, the island 'is a securely anchored aircraft carrier at the intersection point of the lines of tension of the great nuclear powers'.[101]

At the end of this period, the United States had failed to bring an end to the Cyprus problem. Its contribution was directed mainly through the Greek military regime, but failed to bring peace. However, in containing the conflict and preventing its escalation it was successful.

The Soviet Union. The Soviet Union's impact on peacemaking in Cyprus in the 1965-July 1974 period was indirect. Its superpower status offered Greek Cypriots and Turkey an alternative to the United States, which in turn had a negative impact on US policy towards Cyprus: its mere existence in the context of the Cold War, in other words, affected international peacemaking in Cyprus in the above period. The latter was secondary to the Soviets' global aims and Moscow's focus was on the same two principles as before the crisis of 1963-4. One was to maintain the independence and non-alignment of Cyprus, and the other was to disrupt the NATO alliance on its south-eastern flank. Its warning in 1964 against any invasion of Cyprus sustained the first aim and paved the way towards the second. The Soviets condemned the London conference of 1964, and warned the West against interfering in the internal affairs of Cyprus, arguing that safeguarding its independence was the responsibility of the Security Council.[102] They also opposed any intervention by NATO in Cyprus.[103]

The Soviets received Turkey's initiatives for better relations in the early half of the 1960s with enthusiasm, well aware of the strategic importance of the Bosphorus to their growing naval presence in the Indian Ocean and Africa. A series of visits between the top officials of the two countries indicated a shared willingness to establish closer cooperation. From 1965 to 1970 the amount of trade between the two countries quadrupled.[104] The primary aim of this rapprochement for the Soviets was to drive a wedge between Turkey and NATO, and this effect quickly became evident when in December 1965, the Soviet Union along with fifty-four other countries abstained on UN Resolution 2077 (XX) calling on all states to respect the independence and territorial integrity of the Republic of Cyprus. Earlier, in January 1965, the Soviet foreign minister Andhrei Gromyko had issued a statement in which, besides pledging support for the independence, territorial integrity, non-alignment and demilitarisation of Cyprus, he stated: 'They [the Cypriots] may choose the federal form. And this assumes the existence of a single central government, and a single defence organisation, and a single administrative and judicial mechanism.'[105]

However, despite the warming of Soviet-Turkish relations, Makarios still enjoyed Soviet support for Cyprus's independence. It was true that in March 1967 the discovery of a spy network in Cyprus led to the expulsion of a Soviet embassy attaché and the Aeroflot representative in Nicosia.[106] Nevertheless, both countries realised the advantages of maintaining an amicable relationship: Makarios exploited the relations with the Soviets to counter any Western plot against him, and they were more than willing to accommodate him. Just before the end of the Lisbon conference in 1971, at which Turkey and Greece reportedly came to an agreement over Cyprus, Makarios visited Moscow and informed his hosts of the possible dangers of such an agreement.[107]

The developments of the 1960s in Cyprus made it easier for the Soviet leaders to accommodate their interests. With the Greek coup and the expressed wish of Makarios to find a 'feasible solution', the Soviets found it easier to oppose *Enosis* in any form, particularly in the light of their improved relations with Turkey. In other words, in opposing *Enosis* the Soviets were now fully backed not only by Turkey but also by Makarios. In June 1971 in Moscow, Makarios insisted: 'We will resist any attempt to enforce a solution which will lead to political or geographic partition of our island. Nor will we suffer a limitation on the independence and sovereignty of Cyprus.'[108] The Soviet Union reaffirmed in April of the same year, in a joint statement with Turkey, its 'opposition to *Enosis* in any form, for the safeguarding of the independence, sovereignty and territorial integrity of the Republic of Cyprus...'[109] Unsurprisingly, the regime of the Colonels in Greece was viewed with alarm in Moscow: a Tass communiqué talked of the Colonels 'and their agents in Cyprus...struggling to turn Cyprus into a NATO base, and to eliminate the democratic forces in Cyprus with the same criminal and terrorist methods which they use within Greece'.[110] The intercommunal talks had not gone the way the United States and the Greek military had wished were supported by the Soviets, and in a joint statement during Makarios's visit to Moscow the Cypriot and Soviet leaders wished the talks every success.[111]

Overall, the Soviet policy over Cyprus in the 1965-July 1974 period was to maintain the independence of Cyprus, in which it was completely successful, and at the same time to drive a wedge between Turkey and the Western Alliance, in which it achieved only limited success, as when in 1965 Turkey refused to participate in NATO's multilateral force. The Cypriot communist party AKEL continued to be a powerful political force in the island and was directly controlled by the Soviets,[112] providing them with an important source of leverage. Meanwhile, the United Nations was the only outside organisation which enjoyed Soviet support in trying to bring about a peaceful settlement.

The United Nations. The impact of the UN on peacemaking in Cyprus in the 1965-July 1974 period was significant. First, by sanctioning the extension of UNFICYP's mandate during this period, it made peacemaking efforts possible on the island. Secondly, the intercommunal talks of 1968-July 1974 were held under UN auspices, and the good offices of the Secretary-General were used by the UN towards peacemaking efforts. However, these were largely ineffective, owing to the degree of intercommunal mistrust in Cyprus and the opposing aims of the UN and the United States.

Turkey's rejection in 1965 of the Galo Plaza report led to the resignation of the UN mediator, whom the Turks alleged had exceeded his mandate by assuming the role of arbitrator. Henceforth the Turks rejected the notion of a UN mediator for Cyprus,[113] and its mediation efforts – as required by Paragraph 7 of Security Council Resolution 186 – effectively came to an end.[114] It was clearly impractical to keep having to make a new appointment every time one of the parties objected to the mediator's recommendations.[115] And since Plaza's recommendations were clearly different from, if not actually opposed to, those of Acheson, it can be assumed that US policy-makers were not keen to repeat the experience. None of the subsequent resolutions of the Security Council, though reaffirming its Resolution 186, made any direct reference to the appointment of a new mediator.

Although the interested parties in the Cyprus conflict eventually resorted to the UN, they did so for different reasons. By pointing out in its Resolution 186 that a settlement to the conflict had to be sought, the Security Council implicitly acknowledged that the 1960 Agreements needed modification at the very least, substantiating Makarios's similar claim. As has been pointed out, Makarios gained international support for a 'political revolution' in Cyprus by using the UN as 'an instrument to attain the next goals in the continuing struggle for real and complete independence'.[116]

Moreover, the UN gave legitimacy to the Greek Cypriots through formal resolutions such as General Assembly Resolution 2077 (XX) in December 1965. The newly-independent countries were presented with the Cyprus problem as a case of foreign intervention, and so were sympathetic to Makarios, not wanting to take the political and moral risks involved in legitimising the threat of force against the territorial integrity of a fellow UN member. Nor did they wish to substantiate the kind of minority claims which some of them had to deal with in their own countries.

On the other land, the UN had worked against the interests of Turkey and the Turkish Cypriots. Resolutions 186 of the Security Council and 2077 (XX) of the General Assembly both directly implied that the Greek Cypriot-dominated government in Nicosia was the only one in Cyprus to be internationally recognised. And although General Assembly resolutions are not legally binding, they carry strong political and moral force.[117] Furthermore, the remark of U Thant, the Secretary-General, that the solution of the Cyprus problem was 'first and foremost a matter for the "Cypriot government" '[118] was a blow to Turkey and the Turkish Cypriots. Of course, the dispatching of UNFICYP was some form of consolation because it deterred the Greek Cypriots from using their military superiority on the ground against the Turkish Cypriots, but even this was limited as the 1967 crisis showed: some went further in regarding UNFICYP as totally ineffective. According to one Turkish Cypriot observer, the UN's methods of persuasion and negotiation 'only served to prolong the agonies and sufferings of the Turkish Cypriot community'.[119]

The US government had agreed to UN involvement only after all other alternatives had been exhausted, its reluctance being due to the fear that it would formally include the Soviets as a factor in the dispute and give them unwelcome leverage.[120] For its part the Soviet Union supported UN involvement since it highlighted the differences among the Western allies, closed the door to any NATO-based solution and allowed it to veto any solution not to its liking. Thus, the UN had become the only forum through which all the parties concerned, with the exception of Turkey and the Turkish Cypriots, were prepared to pursue their interests. The establishment of UNFICYP was a positive development for all the permanent members of the Security Council and is agreed to have served all their interests.[121]

However, beyond this there was a divergence of interests which the first UN mediation attempt, culminating in the Galo Plaza Report, failed to accommodate. Succeeding UN efforts became more of a formality, passive rather than active. In 1966 U Thant appointed A. Bernardes as his special representative in Cyprus with a broad mandate to make any approaches to the parties that might lead to discussions at any level.

In its Resolution 244 of 22 December 1967 the Security Council invited the parties to avail themselves of the Secretary-General's good offices.

Both these Resolutions clearly coincided with Makarios's views, as the UN could not go against its own Charter: Cyprus was entitled to all the privileges of a member-state, including sovereignty and territorial integrity. However, this did not amount to a blank cheque for the Greek Cypriots; during their economic blockade of the Turkish Cypriots, U Thant said of the restrictions that 'in some instances [they] have been so severe as to amount to a veritable seige, [indicating] that the Government of Cyprus seeks to force a potential solution by economic pressure as a substitute for military action'.[22]

But why did the UN fail to achieve a settlement in the 1965-July 1974 period? The crisis of November 1967 showed up one particular weakness in UNFICYP's mandate in dealing with violence on the island. According to UN records, during the fighting

> UNFICYP observation posts were not bypassed; instead, the National Guard took up positions at or alongside UNFICYP observations posts, thus drawing fire on them. In addition, there were incidents of deliberate damage to UNFICYP equipment and manhandling of UNFICYP personnel by the National Guard. Orally on 15 November and in writing the next day, the Secretary-General protested to the Cyprus Government about the abusive treatment of UNFICYP personnel.[123]

Its ability to use force only for self-defence made the presence of UNFICYP a weak deterrent to the communities in Cyprus and militated against an effective ending of hostilities, which would be needed for success in mediation.

The UN's effectiveness and credibility was also seriously undermined by the parallel mediatory efforts of the United States, whose interests pulled in a different direction. The United States did not object to the Turkish rejection of the Plaza report, and in 1965 voted against General Assembly Resolution 2077 (XX), which was a blow to the UN. Such progress as was eventually made in the intercommunal talks in the aftermath of the 1967 crisis, which never bore fruit, was due not to the work of the UN but rather to the growing sense of political realism of the Greek Cypriot leaders.[124] U Thant's repeated messages[125] to Makarios to expedite the talks were at most ineffective reminders.

Another mounting problem was the deficit over UNFICYP, which ultimately had to be financed by the West, and US pressure to cut the number of personnel in the force: the freezing of the situation had seemed to work to the advantage of Makarios and so a reduction in the force could, in the view of US officials, induce the Greek Cypriots to grant some concessions. These considerations made Cyprus a heavy political and economic burden for the UN.[126]

One should also bear in mind the preventive nature of UN peacemaking and peacekeeping efforts. The peacekeeping role was generally successful, with the exception that it failed to bring about the 'return to normal conditions' prescribed in Security Council Resolution 186. As for the UN's peacemaking role, it offered an official and acceptable framework within which all parties could openly participate. It is noteworthy that only four years after the Plaza report was issued, the 1968-July 1974 intercommunal talks began to bridge the gap between the two communities, exactly in line with one of the Report's recommendations, namely that a solution had to be found 'from within' rather than from outside.

It should also not go unnoticed here that the UN actually called for the designation of a mediator as early as March 1964. This was a significant development as, in the words of Van Coufoudakis, it acknowledged that

> ...peacekeeping is neither identical nor necessarily conducive to peacemaking. The Council's peacekeeping and mediation proposals provided for both the preventive and the therapeutic function. Resolution 186 therefore tacitly recognised the dissatisfaction expressed by many states about UNEF, that without an active mediation effort UNEF had contributed mainly to the pacific perpetuation of the dispute.[127]

Coufoudakis substantiates his claim with examples of the 1967 six day war in the Middle East, and the 1967 and 1974 crises in Cyprus.[128] Also, in establishing UNFICYP, the UN proved its versatility and flexibility at a time when there was a serious battle within the organisation about the application of Article 19 of the UN Charter.[129]

Despite the appointment on 20 February 1967 of a new UN representative, Bibiano F. Osorio-Tafall, the UN's mediatory efforts were dormant in the aftermath of the Plaza report, particularly from 1968 to 1974.[130] During this time the UN's basic role was for the Security Council to receive the periodic reports of the Secretary-General, hold debates on the occasion of renewal of UNFICYP's mandate and emergency sessions such as those during the November-December 1967 crisis, and to reaffirm its basic Resolution 186 and subsequent resolutions.[131] However, it did succeed in making the use of force against the Cyprus state much more difficult. As stated by Coufoudakis,

> This phase of the Cyprus question pointed at the organisation's ability to provide a flexible response to an international crisis, at a difficult time in the life of the UN itself. It also indicated the limits of its peacekeeping and peacemaking capability at a time of minimum

> consensus among the superpowers, and a relative divergence in the goals pursued by the United Nations and the United States in the Cyprus dispute.'[32]

The crisis of November 1967 was successfully contained and a Greco-Turkish war prevented, largely because the United States applied enough pressure on all parties – mainly Greece and Turkey – to reach some kind of agreement before it got out of hand. However the intercommunal talks that took place as a result between 1968 and July 1974 failed to produce any results, reaching deadlock over the extent of the autonomy and authority of the local government. Neither community was prepared to grant enough concessions.

The Greek Cypriots suspected the Turkish Cypriots of harbouring partitionist plans, while the Turkish Cypriots thought the Greek Cypriots still aimed for *Enosis*. The Greek Cypriot leadership's determination to class the Turkish Cypriots as a minority was a further stumbling block. During this period pressure was exerted by Greece on the Greek Cypriots to compromise, but there was no corresponding pressure on the Turkish Cypriots from Turkey.

Finally, the divergence of goals between the United States and the UN reduced the chances of a successful outcome. Support from the United States, as the leader of the Western camp, for the UN's peacemaking role in Cyprus was essential, and the disparity in their mediatory efforts undermined the UN's peacemaking ability in Cyprus. Overall the 1965-July 1974 era was a period when the chances of a settlement to the Cyprus problem were at their best. Regrettably they were not taken.

NOTES

1. Thomas Ehrlich, *International Crises and the Role of Law: Cyprus, 1958-1967*, Oxford University Press, 1974, p. 91.
2. Pierre Oberling, *The Road to Bellapaise: The Turkish Cypriot Exodus to Northern Cyprus*, New York: Social Science Monographs, Boulder, 1982, p. 138.
3. Personal interview with Glafkos Clerides, 14 March 1990.
4. *UN Annual Records*, 1967, p. 278.
5. For an elaborate account of the 1968-July 1974 intercommunal talks see Polyvios G. Polyviou, *Cyprus: Conflict and Negotiation 1960-1980*, London: Duckworth, 1980; see also Glafkos Clerides, *Cyprus: My Deposition*, Nicosia: Alithia Publishing, 1989, volume 2, p. 195.
6. Zaim M. Necatigil, *The Cyprus Question and the Turkish Position in International Law*, Oxford University Press, 1989, p. 63.
7. Polyviou, op. cit., p. 62.
8. Clerides, vol. 2, op. cit., p. 248.

9. Ibid., p. 264.
10. Ibid., p. 273.
11. Ibid., p. 275.
12. Ibid., p. 308.
13. Ibid., p. 309.
14. Ibid., p. 310.
15. Ibid., p. 310.
16. Ibid., pp. 346 and 347.
17. Glafkos Clerides, *Cyprus: My Deposition*, op. cit., vol. 3, 1990, p. 70.
18. Quoted by Michael Attalides, *Cyprus: Nationalism and International Politics*, Edinburgh: Q Press, 1979, p. 102.
19. Necati Munir Ertekun, *In Search of a Negotiated Cyprus Settlement*, Nicosia: n.p., 1981, p. 25.
20. Attalides, op. cit., p. 100.
21. See ibid., p. 101.
22. Quoted by Clerides, vol. 2, op. cit., p. 239.
23. Ibid., p. 382.
24. Ibid., p. 324.
25. Nectati Ertekun, *The Cyprus Dispute and the Birth of the Turkish Republic of Northern Cyprus*, Nicosia: K. Rustem & Bro., 2nd edn, 1984, p. 26.
26. P. Polyviou, *Cyprus in Search of a Constitution*, Nicosia: Nicolaou & Sons, 1976; particularly part II, chapter IV.
27. Ehrlich, op. cit., p. 95.
28. Clerides, vol. 2, op. cit., p. 195.
29. Ibid., p. 205.
30. Ibid., p. 208.
31. *Secretary-General's Report*, Doc. no. S/6569, 29 July 1965.
32. *20 UN SCOR*, 1234th meeting 17 (1965).
33. Markides, *The Rise and Fall of the Cyprus Republic*, New Haven: Yale University Press, 1977, p. 129.
34. Michael Harbottle, 'Why Cyprus is Doomed to Become a Political Volcano', *The Times*, London, 17 October 1974.
35. Markides, op. cit., p. 130.
36. Clerides, vol. 2, op.cit., p. 368.
37. *Secretary-General's Report*, Doc. no. S/10664, 26 May 1972, paras 30 and 58.
38. Clerides, vol. 2, op. cit., p. 324.
39. Clerides, vol. 3, op. cit., p. 263.
40. Clerides, vol. 2, op. cit., p. 382.
41. Ibid., p. 380.
42. Poliviou, *Cyprus: Conflict*, p. 36.
43. Metin Tamkoc, *The Turkish Cypriot State: The Embodiment of the Right of Self-determination*, Nicosia: K. Rustem & Bro., 1988, p. 78.
44. Statement Made Before the Special Political Committee of the General Assembly, October 29, 1974, A/SPC/PV, 922, p. 32.
45. Stanley Kyriakides, *Cyprus: Constitutionalism and Crisis Government*, Philadelphia: University of Pennsylvania Press, 1968, p. 115.
46. Richard A. Patrick, *Political Geography and the Cyprus Conflict, 1963-1971*, Waterloo, Ontario: Dept. of Geography, publication series no. 4, University of Waterloo, 1976, p. 108.
47. *UN Doc.* S/7191, 10 March 1966, paragraph 91.
48. Rauf R. Denktash, *The Cyprus Triangle*, Nicosia: K. Rustem & Bro., 2nd edn 1988, p. 58.
49. Zenon Stavrinides, *The Cyprus Conflict: National Identity and Statehood*, Nicosia: Loris Stavrinides Press, p. 56.

50. Ertekun, *The Cyprus Dispute*, pp. 22 and 28.
51. Oberling, op. cit., p. 123.
52. George W. Ball, *The Past has another Pattern*, New York: W.W. Norton, 1982, p. 348.
53. Richard Crossman, *The Diaries of a Cabinet Minister*, London: Hamish Hamilton/Jonathan Cape, 1976, vol. II, p. 449.
54. *The Guardian*, 2 April 1988.
55. Clerides, vol. 2, op. cit., p. 186.
56. Ibid., p. 328.
57. Ibid., pp. 328-9.
58. Ibid., p. 176.
59. *Cyprus Mail*, 4 and 7 December 1966.
60. Clerides, vol. 2, op. cit., p. 259.
61. Ibid., p. 176.
62. *The Guardian*, 7 September 1967.
63. *New York Times*, 9 May 1965.
64. Ehrlich, op. cit., p. 94.
65. Cited by Attalides, *Cyprus: Nationalism*, p. 131.
66. Sharon Anderholm Weiner, 'Turkish Foreign Policy Decision Making on the Cyprus Issue: A Comparative Analysis of Three Crises', unpubl. Ph.D. thesis, Duke University, 1980, p. 152.
67. Clerides, vol. 2, op. cit., p. 194.
68. Van Coufoudakis, 'United States Foreign Policy and the Cyprus Question: A Case Study in Cold War Diplomacy' in Michael Attalides (ed.), *Cyprus Reviewed*, Nicosia: Jus Cypri Association, 1977, p. 125.
69. *Milliyet*, 30 May 1971 (translation provided by Reza Dehghan).
70. Noted by Attalides, *Cyprus: Nationalism*, p. 134
71. Polyviou, Cyprus: *Conflict*, p. 68.
72. Interview with Laurence Stern, quoted by L. Stern, *The Wrong Horse: The Politics of Intervention and the Failure of American Diplomacy*, New York: Times Books, 1977, p. 106.
73. Attalides, *Cyprus: Nationalism*, p. 133.
74. Polyviou, *Cyprus in Search*, p. 197.
75. Noted by Attalides, *Cyprus: Nationalism*, p. 129.
76. Stephen Ryan, 'Ethnic Conflict and the International System: Foreign Involvement in the Cyprus Problem 1974-1982', unpubl. Ph.D. thesis, London School of Economics, 1984, p. 151.
77. Ferioz Ahmed, *The Turkish Experiment in Democracy: 1960-1975*, London: Hurst, 1977, p. 406.
78. Michael Harbottle, *The Impartial Soldier*, Oxford University Press, 1970, p. 101.
79. Patrick, op. cit., p. 108.
80. Oberling, op. cit., p. 142.
81. Ibid., p. 123.
82. Quoted in *UN Doc*. No. S/8248, 16 November 1967.
83. Tamkoc, op. cit., p. 94.
84. See Attalides, *Cyprus: Nationalism*, p. 98.
85. Necatigil, op. cit., p. 65.
86. Clerides, vol. 2, op. cit., p. 266.
87. Ibid., p. 355.
88. Coufoudakis, op. cit., p. 117.
89. For more details see Coufoudakis, op. cit., p. 141, note 83.
90. Ertekun, *The Cyprus Dispute*, appendix 17, p. 231.
91. Quoted by Christopher Hitchens, *Cyprus*, London: Quartet, 1984, p. 157.

92. For a more elaborate account and more details see Andreas Papandreou, *Democracy at Gunpoint*, Garden City: Doubleday, 1970.
93. US Congress, *Controlling the Damage: US Policy Options for Greece*. Report of a study mission to Greece, 18 to 21 January 1974, Washington, DC, US Government Printing Office, 1974.
94. Attalides, *Cyprus: Nationalism*, p. 130.
95. Coufoudakis, op. cit., p. 123.
96. Adams and Cottrell, *Cyprus Between East and West*, Baltimore: Johns Hopkins University Press, 1968, p. 69.
97. Coufoudakis, op. cit., p. 128.
98. UNFICYP had been reduced by 50% from its initial strength of 6,500 men by December 1972.
99. Van Coufoudakis, 'United Nations Peacekeeping and Peacemaking and the Cyprus Question', *Western Political Quarterly*, 29, 3, 1976, p. 466.
100. Clerides, vol. 2, op. cit., p. 319.
101. Adalbert Weinstein, 'Zyperns Strategische Bedeutung', *Frankfurter Allgemeine Zeitung*, 19 July 1974, quoted by Attalides in *Cyprus: Nationalism*, op. cit., p. 149.
102. Adams and Cottrell, op. cit., p. 35.
103. Coufoudakis, 'United States Foreign Policy', p. 112.
104. Attalides, *Cyprus: Nationalism*, p. 144.
105. Ibid., p. 142.
106. Oberling, op. cit., p. 124.
107. Quoted by Attalides, *Cyprus: Nationalism*, p. 155.
108. Ibid.
109. Ibid., p. 143.
110. Ibid.
111. Ibid., p. 145.
112. Personal interview with Mr Triandaphylides, Attorney General of Cyprus, January 1989.
113. Joseph S. Joseph, 'The UN as an Instrument of National Policy: The Case of Cyprus', *The Cyprus Review*, Nicosia: Intercollege; Indiana: University of Indianapolis, Fall 1989, vol. 1, no. 2, p. 56.
114. Andreas J. Jacovides, 'The Cyprus Problem and the United Nations' in Attalides (ed.), *Cyprus Reviewed*, op. cit., p. 188.
115. Clerides, vol. 3, op. cit., p. 216.
116. See Joseph, op. cit., p. 54.
117. F.C. Ikle, *How Nations Negotiate*, New York: Harper and Row, 1964, p. 21.
118. Ertekun, *The Cyprus Dispute*, p. 19.
119. Tamkoc, op. cit., p. 93.
120. Ball, op. cit., p. 340.
121. Coufoudakis, 'United Nations Peacekeeping', p. 464.
122. *UN Doc*. S/5950, 10 September 1964, para. 222.
123. *UN Annual Records*, 1967, p. 278.
124. Coufoudakis, 'United Nations Peacekeeping', p. 467.
125. Clerides, vol. 2, op. cit., p. 312.
126. *See UN Doc*. S/11137, 1 December 1973, p. 23.
127. Coufoudakis, 'United Nations Peacekeeping', p. 465.
128. Ibid.
129. See John G. Stoessinger, *The United Nations and the Superpowers: China, Russia and America*, New York: Random House, 3rd edn, 1973, pp. 67-126 and 193-201.
130. Jacovides, op. cit., p. 189.
131. Ibid., p. 188.
132. Coufoudakis, 'United Nations Peacekeeping', p. 469.

5

INTERNATIONAL PEACEMAKING IN CYPRUS, JULY 1974-1980

An outline survey

The July 1974-80 period saw an intensification of international peacemaking in Cyprus as events in July and August 1974 again threatened security in the eastern Mediterranean and the cohesion of NATO. The UN undertook a more active role during this period, and a major independent initiative was also launched by the US, British and Canadian governments in 1978. In 1977 and in 1979 two major agreements were reached between the leaders of the two Cypriot communities, but to this day they remain unimplemented. Although international peacemaking during this period failed to bring about a settlement, important developments led to changes of attitude in the two communities that affected the peacemaking process.

The coup and the invasion

The events of 1974 were undoubtedly a turning-point for Cyprus. The Greek-staged coup and the subsequent Turkish invasion left their mark on every aspect of the Cyprus problem, and they altered the framework within which a solution was to be sought. The attitudes of all interested parties were affected by these events, and the process of peacemaking also altered substantially. The coup and the invasion are not in themselves the focus of this chapter, but in as much as they represent the failure of international peacemaking in Cyprus and affect it, their significance is discussed.

On 2 July 1974 Makarios wrote a letter to the Greek President Ghizikis accusing him and the military junta in Greece of supporting, financing and directing the terrorist activities of EOKA-B in Cyprus. The letter, which was printed in the Cyprus press four days later, contained a number of striking statements. For example, it said that it was from Athens

> ....that the tree of evil, the bitter fruits of which the Greek Cypriots are tasting today, is being fed and maintained and helped to grow

> and spread. In order to be absolutely clear, I say that the cadres of the military regime of Greece support and direct the activities of the EOKA-B terrorists...[1]

Makarios was also candid on another matter:

> I have more than once so far felt, and in some cases I have almost touched, a hand invisibly extending from Athens and seeking to liquidate my human existence.[2]

On 5 July the Greek-Cypriot daily *Apogevmatini* (Afternoon) published an editorial that forecast the details of the impending events on the island with remarkable accuracy.[3] On 15 July, these predictions began to materialise as a Greek-staged military coup in Cyprus overthrew the government and seized power. Nikos Sampson, renowned for his dislike of the Turks, was installed as the new president. Makarios had a lucky escape and with British help fled the country.

The subsequent Turkish military invasion of the island, which began on 20 July, was also not altogether unexpected. P.G. Polyviou writes:

> Cyprus in June and July of 1974 was filled with rumours of an impending coup...and in addition evidence was now accumulating that Turkish and Turkish Cypriot forces were being put on a military alert, in expectation no doubt of what in many quarters was now regarded as an inevitable attempt by the Greek regime to overthrow Makarios that would at last provide Turkey with the long awaited opportunity to invade the island.[4]

On 14 August 1974 the second phase of the Turkish invasion began in Cyprus, leading to considerable human suffering. Turkey occupied about one-third of the island and started to expel Greek Cypriots from the occupied north to the south. In December 1974 Makarios returned and resumed the post of president, which in his absence had been filled by Glafkos Clerides.

After the invasion, negotiations with the Turkish Cypriots had to be conducted within a different framework. The military presence of Turkey in the north of the island now meant that the Turkish Cypriots would enter any dialogue with their fellow Greek Cypriots from a position of strength and would naturally do their utmost to take advantage of it at the negotiating table. However, the first attempt at peacemaking in the aftermath of the Turkish invasion was the Geneva talks between the guarantor powers.

The Geneva talks

First round, 25-30 July 1974. Following the Greek-staged coup and the Turkish invasion, the UN Security Council called on Britain, Greece and Turkey to enter negotiations without delay for the restoration of peace and the constitutional government in Cyprus (Resolution 353 of 20 July 1974, paragraph 5). On 22 July 1974 the British foreign secretary James Callaghan announced in the House of Commons that Turkey and Greece had accepted his invitation for peace talks in Geneva.[5] The actual negotiations began on 25 July and lasted for five days. On 30 July the British, Greek and Turkish foreign ministers – Callaghan, Mavros and Gunes – agreed that the areas already controlled by each side in Cyprus were not to be extended and that all hostilities were to cease. A security zone was to be established which only UNFICYP could enter. Greek Cypriots agreed to evacuate all Turkish Cypriot enclaves occupied by them, and to exchange or release hostages. But perhaps the most important provisions in the agreement concerned the acknowledgement of two separate administrations in Cyprus, those of Greek Cypriots and Turkish Cypriots. The difficulties raised by the existence of these parallel administrations were to be considered in the second round of the talks.[6]

Second round of the Geneva talks, 8-14 August 1974. The second round of the Geneva talks started on 8 August 1974 'in an atmosphere of charges and countercharges'.[7] Mutual accusations of violations of the ceasefire by the Greeks and the Turks embittered the initial stages, but despite this early setback the talks proceeded with a certain degree of optimism on the part of Callaghan and the US observer, Hartmann.[8] The representatives of Greece, Turkey, Britain and the UN agreed on a demarcation line separating the two warring factions,[9] while the Greek Cypriot representative Glafkos Clerides, the Turkish Cypriot representative Rauf Denktash, and the Turkish representative Gunes put forward separate plans for a settlement. The basic difference between the two sides – Greece and the Greek Cypriots on the one hand and Turkey and the Turkish Cypriots on the other – was whether the 1960 constitution could be accepted as the legal document on which negotiations could be based. While Greece and the Greek Cypriots claimed it as the point of reference in the negotiations, Turkey and the Turkish Cypriots argued that it had proved unworkable and should be abandoned.[10]

However, negotiations eventually failed when the Turkish side proposed a federation to give Turkish Cypriots autonomy and a cantonal system that would allow them to administer a smaller area.[11] When Clerides asked for thirty-six hours to consider the Turkish proposals, he received a strongly negative answer from Gunes, which led to the collapse of the talks. According to Callaghan, at 2.25 a.m. on the morning of 14 August 'Gunes rose from the table at which we sat, ungracious as ever, and departed, followed by his aides.'[12] The Turkish foreign minister immediately phoned his prime minister, Ecevit, and with the codeword 'My daughter is going on vacation'[13] gave the go-ahead for the second phase of the invasion. And so at 4.30 a.m. on 14 August 1974 the second Turkish military operation against Cyprus began.

The Vienna Talks

In February 1975 the Turkish Cypriot leadership announced the establishment of a 'Turkish Federated State of Cyprus' in the area controlled by the Turkish army. The Security Council, in Resolution 367 adopted on 12 March 1975, asked for a resumption of the talks and as a result five rounds of negotiations known as the Vienna talks took place.

First Round, 28 April-3 May 1975. During the first round, one open and eight closed meetings were held. The representatives of the two communities were Glatkos Clerides for the Greek Cypriot side and Rauf Denktash for the Turkish Cypriot side. All the meetings were held under the chairmanship of the UN Secretary-General, Kurt Waldheim. The powers and functions of the central government, the question of displaced persons and the geographical aspects of a possible settlement in Cyprus formed the basis of negotiations. Perhaps the only notable agreement during the first round was an accord on the reopening of Nicosia's international airport,[14] which to this day remains unimplemented.

Second round of the Vienna talks, 5-7 June 1975. This round consisted of three meetings between the two sides. The main issue was that of the powers and functions of the federal government, which was problematic since the Greek Cypriots preferred to discuss territory first and then move on to the powers of the central government, while the Turkish Cypriots wanted to discuss the central government before other topics.[15] The possibility of a transitional government was also suggested and the two sides agreed to examine the suggestion.[16] However, the UN Secretary-General stated that despite frank discussions the problem remained to be solved.[17]

Third round of Vienna talks, 31 July-2 August 1975. Four meetings were held during the third round of the Vienna Talks and a number of agreements were reached. According to a press communiqué, these included *inter alia*:[18]

(1) The Turkish Cypriots at present in the South of the Island will be allowed, if they want to do so, to proceed North with their belongings under an organized programme and with the assistance of UNFICYP.

(2) Mr Denktash reaffirmed, and it was agreed, that the Greek Cypriots at present in the North of the Island are free to stay and that they will be given every help to lead a normal life, including facilities for education and for the practice of their religion, as well as medical care by their own doctors and freedom of movement in the North.

Other provisions related to the well-being of the members of the two communities trapped in the territory of the opposite side. The question of territory and the powers and functions of the central government were also discussed in this round. Denktash agreed to submit proposals by the end of August, to be discussed between him and Clerides before the start of the fourth round of the talks.

Fourth round of the Vienna talks, 8-10 September 1975. This round, held in New York, reached a stalemate as Denktash failed to submit the concrete proposals that had been agreed in the previous round. Also it appeared that the Turkish Cypriots were not now prepared to stand by agreements reached during previous rounds of the Talks.

Fifth round of the Vienna Talks, 17-21 February 1976. The two most contentious issues of the Cyprus problem, the territorial aspect and the powers and functions of the central government, predominated in this round of the talks. It was agreed to exchange proposals, and this took place in April 1976. While the Greek-Cypriot proposals asked for a central government, the Turkish Cypriot plans called for a weak federal government with increased powers for the federated states.[19] Neither of these proposals found favour.

The Makarios-Denktash High-Level Agreement, 1977

Following the failure of the Vienna talks, a meeting was arranged between Makarios and Denktash on 27 January 1977 in the presence of the Secretary-General's special representative in Cyprus, Javier Pérez de Cuéllar, at the UN headquarters in Nicosia. This was the first time the two leaders had met in fourteen years. In a subsequent meeting between them on 12 February 1977, a four-point Agreement was reached which was to be the basis for future negotiations. The points in the agreement were as follows:[20]

(1) We are seeking an independent, Non-Aligned bicommunal Federal Republic.
(2) The territory under the administration of each community should be discussed in the light of economic viability or productivity and land ownership.
(3) Questions of principle, like freedom of movement, freedom of settlement, the right of property and other specific matters, are open for discussion, taking into consideration the fundamental basis of a bicommunal federal system and certain practical difficulties which may arise for the Turkish Cypriot community.

(4) The powers and functions of the central federal government will be such as to safeguard the unity of the country, having regard to the bicommunal character of the State.

This agreement was significant, since it laid down the guidelines for future negotiations between the two communities.

Second series of Vienna Talks, 31 March-7 April 1977

During the second series of the Vienna Talks the Greek Cypriots submitted proposals on the territorial aspect of the problem and the Turkish Cypriots on the constitutional aspect. The Greek Cypriot plans included provisions to maintain the undivided sovereignty of the island and to protect the rights to property, freedom to move and settle throughout the country. The Turkish Cypriot proposals called for the establishment of a federal government based on the equality of the two communities. The functions of the federal government would grow in time, in what was referred to by Turkish Cypriots as a 'federation by evolution'. However, Greek Cypriots claimed that the Turkish Cypriot proposals would lead to confederation rather than federation, and would further separate the two communities, while the Turkish Cypriots asserted that the Greek Cypriot plans lacked the elements of bi-zonality and economic viability and, if adopted, would deprive the Turkish Cypriot community of vital resources.[21]

The Kyprianou-Denktash High-Level Agreement of 1979

Notwithstanding the hard line that the two communities' leaders had adopted, on 19 May 1979 a ten-point Agreement was reacted between President Kyprianou (who had succeeded Makarios after his unexpected death in 1977) and Denktash. The Agreement was the result of two days of intense negotiations chaired by the UN Secretary-General, and consisted of the following ten points:[22]

(1) Intercommunal talks will resume on 15 June 1979.
(2) The basis for the talks will be the Makarios/Denktash guidelines of 12 February 1977 and the United Nations resolutions relevant to the Cyprus question.
(3) There should be respect for the human rights and fundamental freedoms of all citizens of the Republic.
(4) The talks will deal with all territorial and constitutional aspects.
(5) Priority will be given to reaching agreement on the resettlement of Varosha [the mainly Greek Cypriot part of Famagusta] under United Nations auspices simultaneously with the beginning of consideration by the interlocutors of the constitutional and territorial aspects of a comprehensive settlement. After agreement on Varosha has been reached, it will be implemented without awaiting the outcome of the discussion on other aspects of the Cyprus problem.

(6) The parties will abstain from any action which might jeopardize the outcome of the talks, and special importance will be given to initial practical measures by both sides to promote goodwill, mutual confidence and a return to normal conditions.
(7) The demilitarisation of the Republic of Cyprus is envisaged, and matters relating thereto will be discussed.
(8) The independence, sovereignty, territorial integrity and non-alignment of the Republic should be adequately guaranteed against union in whole or in part with any other country and against any form of partition or secession.
(9) The intercommunal talks will be carried out in a continuing and sustained manner, avoiding any delay.
(10) The intercommunal talks will take place at Nicosia.

This agreement was a breakthrough and hopes were raised of an eventual solution, but they gradually faded as its terms remained unimplemented.

The American-British-Canadian initiative, 1978

In November 1978 a joint US-UK-Canada Plan was drafted and put to the disputants. It consisted of the following:[23]

(1) Cyprus was to become a 'bi-communal federal state with two constituent regions', one populated mostly by Greeks, the other by Turks. Neither of the regions was to unite with any other state.
(2) The new constitutional structure was to be negotiated on the basis of the Western Framework and Makarios-Denktash Agreement of February 1977, and the relevant UN resolutions.
(3) The new constitution was to include the fundamental rights and liberties of the people of Cyprus.
(4) The federal government was to have power over foreign affairs, external defence, currency and central banking, inter-regional and foreign commerce, communications, federal finance, customs, immigration and civil aviation.
(5) The legislative power of the federal government was to be exercised by a bicameral legislature, with an upper house composed of the same number of Greek and Turkish Cypriots and a lower house based on the percentage of Greek and Turkish Cypriots in Cyprus. The approval of both houses was to be required for the passing of any bill. If the upper house rejected it, a two-thirds majority in the lower house, provided that 38 per cent of the representatives were present, could override its decision. There was to be a president and a vice-president, one from each community. Jointly they were to appoint a council of ministers, where neither community was to have fewer than 30 per cent of the positions. Also, both of them were to be able to jointly veto any legislation, but this veto was to be overridden if a two-thirds vote was obtained in both houses. A federal supreme court was to be established, composed of one Greek, one Turk, and one non-Cypriot, and which was to have the power, among other things, to interpret the constitution. Finally, there was to be a fair participation by both communities in the civil service.
(6) The governments of the two regions were to have the powers not vested in the federal government.

(7) An agency was to be created for the purpose of encouraging cooperation between the two communities.
(8) The territory under the authority of each region was to depend on the consideration of such criteria as 'economic viability and productivity, land ownership, security, population patterns and historical factors'. For this purpose, the Turkish Cypriots were to agree on territorial adjustments.
(9) There was to be provision for helping displaced persons return to their regions and for providing compensation for those who did not wish to return.
(10) All non-Cypriot military forces, with the exception of those allowed under the Agreements, were to be withdrawn, and the possibility of the demilitarisation of Cyprus was to be considered.
(11) A reconciliation fund, financed by the federal government and administered by the two regions, was to be established for the purpose of aiding areas needing assistance.
(12) For the purpose of promoting confidence and goodwill between the two communities, the resettlement of Varosha area was to take place under UN auspices.

This plan also failed to win the approval of both communities because the Greek Cypriot side objected to a few of its provisions. Their response will be outlined in greater detail later.

The Greek Cypriot attitude to international peacemaking in Cyprus, July 1974-1980

During the July 1974-80 period, the Greek Cypriots' approach to peacemaking in Cyprus was somewhat confused, but on the whole there was a marked change from previous years. The psychological blow of the Turkish invasion had unsettled the Greek Cypriot leaders and awakened them to some harsh realities. The two High-Level Agreements reached between the two communities in 1977 and 1979 were the manifestation of this changed attitude of the Greek Cypriots, who now accepted federation as the basis of a solution – in itself a big step. However, the mistrust of the Turkish Cypriots prevailed throughout this period, as the Greek Cypriots were wary of partition with some 40,000 Turkish troops stationed in the northern part of the island. As before, the political life of the Greek Cypriots and the Republic of Cyprus continued to be dominated by Makarios up to his death in 1977: any peacemaking initiative depended for success on his blessing.

The Turkish invasion and the horrific human suffering it left in its wake had a sobering effect on Greek Cypriot society, and ended any hope of achieving *Enosis*. For Makarios, the independence and non-alignment of Cyprus, together with the majority status of the Greek Cypriots, remained essential to any settlement.[24] However, this majority-minority concept[25] was now increasingly questioned by Greek Cypriots and sometimes even dismissed as a dream. In a speech on 6 November

1974, Acting-President Clerides described as an illusion the belief among the Greek Cypriots before the Turkish invasion 'that we could treat the Turkish Cypriot community as a simple minority, without taking into account that it was backed by Turkey with a population of 33 million.'[26]

Another effect of the invasion on the Greek Cypriots was that it fostered a rapid growth of mistrust of the West in general and of the United States in particular. Greek Cypriots thought it inconceivable that Turkey could have invaded Cyprus without the consent or acquiescence of the West. By blaming the West, Greek Cypriots were, in the words of one commentator, 'able to avoid having to revise their basic political convictions, or raise any deeper questions concerning their traditional relations to the Turks and President Makarios' policies since 1960'.[27] This was negative thinking in two ways. First it ignored the past mistakes and attitudes of the Greek Cypriot leadership, and secondly it promoted the view that any future solution initiated by the West would probably favour the Turkish Cypriots rather than them and was therefore not worth considering.

The Turkish invasion also deprived the Greek Cypriots of two important levers, turning the military advantage in favour of the Turkish Cypriots, and providing the Turkish Cypriot leadership with the authority, sanctioned during the Vienna Talks,[28] to gather all its population in the north, separated from the Greek Cypriots – so much so that by September 1975 only 130 Turkish Cypriots remained in the south[29] and by the end of November 1981 only 1,076 Greek Cypriots lived in the occupied northern part.[30]

With the return of Makarios to the island on 7 December 1974, and his immediate reinstatement as President of the Republic, sharp differences emerged between him and Clerides – of which his pronouncement that Clerides had an 'over-enthusiasm for making concessions'[31] was a clear manifestation. Public opinion was on Makarios's side; already before his return, on 29 September 1974 between 25,000 and 30,000 people had turned out to demonstrate their support for him in Limassol. As we have seen, there were a number of factors involved here. Makarios was the leader of the struggle for independence, the first President of the Republic and the Archbishop of Cyprus; he was skillful in his conduct of domestic politics, and possessed personal charisma. And because the Turkish invasion had been a severe psychological blow to the Greek Cypriots in terms of pride and honour,[32] his rhetorical statements satisfied undoubted psychological needs in his people. For instance, he was quoted in a Greek Cypriot newspaper as saying that his signature would 'never be put under an agreement that will give even a stone to the Turks',[33] which was not the sort of remark that Clerides would ever have made.

The public division between Makarios and Clerides had a negative impact on the peacemaking process. Clerides was a politician, trusted by the Turkish Cypriots and by Turkey, whose goodwill could be exploited for peacemaking on the island. On his becoming acting president during Makarios's absence in the aftermath of the coup and the invasion, the Turkish government reacted by stating'This is welcome news'.[34] The Turkish Cypriot leader Denktash also welcomed the news: 'He is satisfactory for us. He is a Cypriot who loves Cyprus and will not deviate into cheating.'[35]

After Makarios's return Clerides resumed his previous position as speaker of the House of Representatives, and was now appointed by Makarios as the Greek Cypriot chief interlocutor in the Vienna talks. Some have attributed his appointment to insistence by the Greek prime minister Constantine Karamanlis and the UN Secretary-General Kurt Waldheim, both of whom were familiar with his rapport with the Turkish Cypriot leaders and his diplomatic skills.[36] Nonetheless, Clerides's position as chief negotiator was not easy, and he tried to resign in January 1976, only to withdraw his resignation after being persuaded by Waldheim and Karamanlis. But when he came under heavy attack in the Greek Cypriot press because of a secret agreement he had made with Denktash in the fifth round of the Vienna talks, he resigned finally on 7 April, three months later. The substance of this agreement had been merely to submit a set of Greek Cypriot proposals ten days earlier than the official deadline in order to give Denktash ample time – and to deprive him of the possible excuse of not having had enough time – to submit concrete proposals of his own. Clerides had been regarded by many, including Secretary-General Waldheim, as the Greek Cypriot leader most likely to reach an agreement[37] with the Turkish Cypriot authorities, and his resignation was a setback.

The most notable impact of the Turkish invasion was that it made the concept of federation an inseparable part of any settlement. The Vienna talks were the forum at which this concept was tied to the negotiations, and it was during these meetings that the Greek Cypriot side showed its willingness to accept federation as a basis for settlement. As acting president Clerides had already announced publicly that he could see 'no prospect of the Turks accepting any settlement that does not include federation';[38] in his view this was 'the only realistic way of settling the island's political crisis'.[39] This was a big enough step and any further concessions to the Turkish Cypriots could have been seen as a humiliating sign of weakness.[40]

The US-British-Canadian Plan proposed in November 1978 was opposed by the Greek Cypriots on all grounds, but especially because of its provision for the extent of federal power, the territorial aspect of the federation, and curtailment of 'freedom of movement', 'freedom of settlement' and 'the right to property'.[41] These three basic freedoms were at the forefront of the Greek Cypriots' demands at the time.

Makarios died of a heart attack on 3 August 1977. In an interview a short time earlier, he admitted he had made mistakes, saying: 'I must say that I am not happy, looking back, on how I acted in some cases'.[42] The death of the charismatic Archbishop, who had dominated Greek Cypriot politics for more than two decades, made no dramatic change in the course of peacemaking in Cyprus. However, despite early calls 'for the preservation of unity on the basis of Makarios's foreign and domestic policies',[43] his death brought Greek Cypriot divisions into the open. Weakened by the lack of unity, Spyros Kyprianou, who succeeded Makarios as head of state by winning the 1978 presidential election, lacked credibility with the Turkish Cypriots, who were sceptical of his ability to live up to any agreement.[44] The new president also took a hard line, which obviously did not help the peacemaking process.

Kyprianou's role in peacemaking with the Turkish Cypriots has been criticised by the Greek Cypriots themselves. In May 1980 Ezekias Papaioannou, the leader of AKEL, complained that he had failed to establish proper contact and dialogue with the Turkish Cypriot opposition to Denktash.[45] In March 1980 Alecos Michaelides, speaker of the House of Representatives, went as far as telling a Turkish newspaper correspondent that there could be no solution to the Cyprus problem as long as Kyprianou remained in power.[46] In November of the same year, Tassos Papadopoulos, who succeeded Clerides in the intercommunal talks for a while and subsequently was himself succeeded by George Ioannides, attacked Kyprianou publicly at a press conference for being autocratic and lacking a precise policy in the intercommunal talks.[47] These deep divisions among the Greek Cypriots weakened their position at the negotiating table, making them incapable of granting any concessions towards a settlement.

As for international support, the Greek Cypriots continued to enjoy the backing of the UN and the Non-Aligned Movement in the July 1974-1980 period, expressed in various UN resolutions. Nevertheless, this support was only verbal, contained in official statements and votes, and could not 'dislodge 40,000 troops and 250 armed vehicles from the north of the island'.[48]

An aggravating problem for the Greek Cypriots was the arrival of a large influx of Turkish settlers from the mainland in the north of the island, changing the overall demographic balance. Turkey, with a population of around 36 million in 1975, could afford to dispatch 'several hundred thousands of impoverished peasants in a short time'.[49] According to some figures in 1977, the number of Turks from the mainland then settled in north Cyprus exceeded 20,000.[50] In time this huge migration could adversely affect the Greek Cypriots' ability to negotiate a settlement; the sooner one was reached, the sooner the influx of Turkish settlers could cease.

In sum, the loss of military superiority put pressure on the Greek Cypriots to reach an agreement with the Turkish Cypriots, since the latter were no longer a weak minority scattered all over the island but rather a strong community concentrated in one geographically cohesive area. International condemnation of the Turkish invasion and global support for the Greek Cypriots seemed to have little effect either on Turkey or on the Turkish Cypriots and in the meantime the influx of Turkish settlers threatened to upset the demographic balance of the island irreversibly. During this period, international recognition of their status as the government of Cyprus and the economic embargo of the Turkish Cypriots were the Greek Cypriots' only bargaining counters, and their attitude became more conciliatory. Nevertheless, the invasion had reinforced their belief that the ultimate aim of the Turkish Cypriots was partition and this fear was reflected in the failure of the Vienna Talks on the issue of territory and the functions and powers of the central government. Overall, however, the Greek Cypriots played a positive role in peacemaking in Cyprus between July 1974 and 1980.

The Turkish Cypriot attitude towards international peacemaking in Cyprus, July 1974-1980

Meanwhile the attitude towards peacemaking of the Turkish Cypriots, with the might of the Turkish army behind them, hardened dramatically. In the aftermath of the invasion, Turkish Cypriot politics were influenced more by Turkey than by Rauf Denktash, who in February 1973 had succeeded Fazil Küchük as the president of the executive committee of the provisional Turkish Cypriot administration, so becoming the new Turkish Cypriot leader. In June 1976, fifteen months after the unilateral declaration of the 'Turkish Federated State of Cyprus' (TFSC) by the Turkish Cypriots, Denktash was formally elected as the leader of his community. However, the main reason for his dominance over Turkish Cypriot affairs was his close ties with Turkey and the fact that he did not deviate from the guidelines set by the mother-country. Turkish pressure on him to accept the return of Makarios to Cyprus in 1974,[51] not to declare an independent state,[52] and to keep the term 'federated' in 'TFSC'[53] was completely effective. The extent of Turkey's influence on Denktash has been described by James Callaghan when recalling the second round of the Geneva conference in 1974, which he attended as British foreign secretary: '[He] was not a free agent, and confessed to me that in the last resort he was obliged to obey his masters on the Turkish mainland.'[54] In fact Denktash, unlike Makarios, was prepared to accept a solution worked out by the two mother-countries.[55] This is not to suggest that he had no say at all in the affairs of his community; for example, he retained his constitutional adviser, Soysal, despite Turkey's desire to remove him.[56] However, the outline of Turkish Cypriot policy, if not actually dictated by Turkey, required its blessing.

Denktash was basically a hardliner for whom the problem was a basic question of security arising from the continued fear of *Enosis*.[57] This was still, in the eyes of the Turkish Cypriot leaders, the root of all evil and the reason for the Greek-staged coup in Cyprus in 1974:[58] the Turkish 'peace operation', as they prefer to call the invasion, was necessary to prevent the realisation of *Enosis*. For Denktash the events of 1974 were a clear manifestation of the failure of the 1960 constitution to serve the interests of his community.[59]

The Greek-staged coup in 1974 was proof to the Turkish Cypriots that without the protection of a new structure their lives and security would always be at the mercy of the Greek Cypriots. 'Federation' was the foundation on which Denktash wanted to base a settlement, and his commitment to this principle was embodied in a statement he issued on 13 February 1975, when the TFSC was unilaterally declared by the Turkish Cypriots. In it he announced the final objective of the TFSC to be 'to unite with the Greek Cypriot community within the framework of a bi-zonal federation'.[60] He also declared his commitment to the independence and non-alignment of Cyprus and stated his opposition to either the union or the partition of the island.[61] His strongest card was the presence of the Turkish troops, which enabled him to negotiate from a position of strength, and led to his making various statements to the effect that the Turkish troops would remain in Cyprus 'for several generations'.[62]

The most important effect of the Turkish invasion on Turkish Cypriots was that it dramatically toughened their stance. Even before the second invasion, during the second round of the Geneva Conference, this change was noticeable in their rejection of Clerides' generous offers of autonomy. According to Oberling:

> Had the proposal been made several years earlier, it would have been warmly received by the Turkish Cypriot leadership as an important step in the right direction. But now it was too little, too late.[63]

Another writer reiterates this view:

> If the Turks had, for more than a decade, stuck it out under virtual conditions of siege, insisting on self-government and independence from the larger Greek community, they are not going to be more moderate now that Jerusalem seems (or seems to their leaders) to be in sight.[64]

The hard stance adopted by Denktash did not, however, mean that he could not reach an understanding with the Greek Cypriots. As James Callaghan recollected,

> There were flashes of common sense [in the second round of the Geneva negotiations]. Acting President Glafkos Clerides and Rauf Denktash, the leader of the Turkish Committee, had brought intelligence and genuine concern to the discussion on the future of their country. If it had been left to them it is conceivable that they might have hammered out an understanding.[65]

On the face of it, therefore, a settlement between the two communities was not out of the question. However, as will be discussed later, the dominance of Turkey over Turkish Cypriots was in many ways conducive to stalemate. The attitude of the Turkish Cypriot leadership towards peacemaking efforts tended to fluctuate. For instance, on 13 April 1978 they issued a set of proposals which the UN Secretary-General praised for dealing with the constitutional and territorial aspects 'in a concrete and substantial way'.[66] Unfortunately, however, this was not the general trend. In a situation requiring the building up of intercommunal confidence and trust, the attitude of the Turkish Cypriot leadership was disappointing. For instance, the UN Secretary-General, in his report to the Security Council on 8 December 1975, criticised the Turkish Cypriots for not taking the necessary measures to help the Greek Cypriots in the north of the country,[67] while the lack of progress in intercommunal talks after Makarios's death has been attributed to the failure of the Turks to produce counter-proposals.[68]

Economically, Turkish Cypriots continued to be in a weaker position than the Greek Cypriots. Although the Turkish invasion brought 70 per cent of the island's economic potential under their control,[69] by January 1978 the cost of living in the occupied north was twice as high as in the south.[70] Their trade deficit in 1980 amounted to over $46 million,[71] and they became heavily dependent on Turkish subsidies for survival.[72] There was also a shortage of badly-needed foreign currency.[73] Another problem for the Turkish Cypriot community was the influx of the Turkish settlers, for although they are basically of the same stock, the Turks from the mainland are different in social conduct and behaviour. The resulting tension between the two groups led Küchük, the former Turkish Cypriot leader, to call on Turkey to withdraw them from Cyprus.[74] In the words of one Turkish Cypriot, 'The troops that have been sent here are a necessary evil. But the 25,000 mainland settlers who have been sent here are not necessary. They're just evil.'[75] The combination of severe economic difficulties and the influx of mainland settlers might have encouraged the Turkish Cypriot leaders to reach a settlement with their fellow islanders, the Greek Cypriots, in this period, but in reality things worked differently. The economic pressures experienced by the Turkish Cypriots tended to increase their dependence on Turkey, which became a negative factor in peacemaking, while the settlers were seen by the Turkish Cypriot leaders as a lever to force concessions out of the Greek Cypriots.

Internationally Turkish Cypriots failed to obtain recognition. Although the eighth world session of the World Muslim Congress was held in northern Cyprus in March 1980, even the Islamic countries did not go so far as to recognise the Turkish Cypriot state.[76] Having failed to obtain international recognition, Denktash protested to the UN Secretary-General at the Greek Cypriots' status. As he put it in one of his letters to the Secretary-General,

> The Republic of Cyprus was established in 1960 as a bi-national state based on the existence of two national communities. [...] Lawful authority in Cyprus is therefore based on the joint will of both the Turkish Cypriot and Greek Cypriot communities, and this authority can neither be assumed nor exercised by either community without the consent of the other.[77]

Internally things did not go well for the Turkish Cypriots either. In 1978-9 there were several cabinet crises, leading to the resignation of eleven deputies from the ruling party, which destroyed its majority in the Turkish Cypriot assembly. Nonetheless, the Turkish Cypriots presented a more unified image than the Greek Cypriots.

In conclusion, the impact of the Turkish invasion on Turkish Cypriots affected peacemaking in Cyprus in a number of ways. First, the establishment of two separate zones, being the direct result of Turkish military action in Cyprus, in effect toughened the stance of Turkish Cypriots, who were no longer in any rush to make concessions.[78] Secondly, the Turkish military presence tightened Ankara's grip on the Turkish Cypriot leadership, reducing its freedom of manoeuvre in negotiations with the Greek Cypriots. Thirdly, the Turkish military operation, which had been automatically supported by the Turkish Cypriots, received international condemnation, putting them at loggerheads with the international community and the United Nations and making peacemaking efforts even harder than before.

The main reason for the failure of peacemaking efforts in the July 1974-80 period, as already stated, was the disagreement over the powers of the central government and the territorial adjustments. While the Greek Cypriots claimed that the Turkish Cypriot proposals would lead to a confederation and not a federation, the Turkish Cypriots maintained that the Greek Cypriot proposals would lead to a unitary state and not a federation.[79] The Turkish Cypriot stance, which had previously changed slightly from time to time, became more inflexible after the

Turkish invasion. In theory, there were incentives for them to come to a settlement with the Greek Cypriots, to rescue their economy and gain the status and legitimacy that Turkey unilaterally could never provide. Yet their continued suspicions of the Greek Cypriots' willingness to treat them as equals made them negative towards peacemaking: their demands increased greatly during this period and despite the High-Level Agreements of 1977 and 1979, they refused to work towards their implementation.

Outside powers and international peacemaking in Cyprus, July 1974-1980

The United Kingdom. The attitude of Britain towards Cyprus after the coup and the Turkish invasion was strongly influenced by United States policy. Although there were differences of opinion between the two, British policy-makers were careful not to deviate from the main policy outlines of the State Department. Britain's peacemaking ability in Cyprus was not fully utilised during this period and there was no independent British initiative.

Both countries adopted a 'do nothing' policy which did little to deter the Turkish army from advancing on Cyprus,[80] in spite of Callaghan's belief that only military intervention would deter it.[81] It has been suggested that if Britain had been prepared to intervene with its own forces between the two sides,[82] the Turkish invasion would have been more limited than it actually was: but for Britain to act unilaterally could have placed it in an uncomfortable position. Callaghan later said he had had 'no intention of exposing Britain to the kind of differences with the United States which existed at the time of the Suez invasion and which had resulted in a terrible setback for British arms and influence'.[83] Britain was no longer a superpower, Callaghan told Clerides during the Geneva talks, and could only act within the context of a UN or American initiative.[84] For Britain, working with the United States and through the United Nations were seen as complementary aspects of a policy to deal with the Cyprus problem. In a personal message to the US Secretary of State Henry Kissinger during the July 1974 crisis, Callaghan said that Britain and America 'should work bilaterally, aiming to bring the parties together, but also using the United Nations for this purpose'.[85] However, in Britain the government's lack of action during the Turkish invasion of Cyprus was very much criticised. A Parliamentary Select Committee Report on Cyprus published on 8 April 1976 complained:

'Britain had a legal right to intervene, she had the moral obligation to intervene, she had the military capacity to intervene. She did not intervene for reasons which the Government refuses to give.'[86]

The government was also criticised for having turned down the Turkish government's request to use the British bases in Cyprus[87] for the invasion which, some argue, might have enabled it to limit the advance of the Turkish army to some extent. However, the government defended its policy[88] arguing, in Callaghan's words, that it had 'behaved honourably and fulfilled its obligations to the limit of the possibilities open to us'.[89]

A key element in British policy was to avoid provoking any of the parties in the conflict and to behave impartially towards both Cypriot communities. This was a difficult task indeed, as an incident in the aftermath of the invasion showed. About 9,000 Turkish Cypriots had taken refuge in the British Akrotiri base during the fighting and Turkey had asked the British government to allow them to be transformed to Turkey so that they could be resettled in north Cyprus. Despite Britain's efforts to transfer this issue to the intercommunal talks, it finally gave in and in 1975 allowed the refugees to leave for Turkey. This greatly upset the Greek Cypriots, and the Cyprus government made an official complaint to the British high commissioner in Nicosia. However, it is believed that Britain complied with the Turkish request only after coming under pressure from its NATO allies, who did not wish to see Turkey antagonised any further.

Britain's main policy at this time was to support the intercommunal talks. Roy Hattersley, minister of state at the Foreign and Commonwealth Office, stated Britain's position as follows: 'Our obligation to reality requires us to hope for, and to promote, the successful outcome of the talks, rather than to mount the initiative on our own.'[90] In the absence of any new initiative, Britain did not engage in consultations over Cyprus with the other guarantor powers. This was confirmed by Ian Gilmour, as principal spokesman for Foreign and Commonwealth Affairs, during a House of Commons debate in January 1980, and he added that there were no plans for any such contacts in the future.[91] Britain's main contribution was to the joint American-British-Canadian Plan in 1978, which the Cyprus government rejected.

All in all, British peacemaking ability in Cyprus between July 1974 and 1980 was not fully utilised. As a guarantor power it had the right, perhaps even the duty, to work towards a settlement. Militarily it was in an ideal position to deter violence on the island through its bases, and it could also have used its close relations with the United States to seek to persuade Washington to involve itself fully in a search for a lasting settlement. At times Britain tried to justify its 'do nothing' policy on the grounds that any action might upset one of the parties and be counterproductive. For instance, in the aftermath of the invasion when the huge influx of Turkish settlers into Cyprus was taking place, the British government refused to criticise Turkey because, according to the then foreign secretary, David Owen, 'it would not help in establishing a better atmosphere if at this stage I were to try to ascribe blame to either side'.[92]

Britain could have tried in two ways to bring about a settlement – by proposing an international conference on Cyprus and by applying pressure on Turkey. However, neither of these would have been viable taking into account the constraints on British policy. An international conference would have given the Soviets a say in any solution, which would probably have exposed Britain to attack from that quarter over its retention of the sovereign base areas in Cyprus. In any case, Soviet involvement would not have been tolerated by the United States. And to apply pressure on Turkey would have risked antagonising a strategically important ally, and possibly weakening its loyalities to the West and NATO.

The most important issue for Britain in Cyprus was of course its use of the Sovereign Bases. And since the government of Cyprus, perhaps because of the Turkish occupation of the north of the country, had shown no signs of wanting to challenge their status, there was no immediate threat to Britain's fundamental interests. However, it should be noted that Britain did support the role of the UN as the international body entrusted with conducting peacemaking functions on the island. Although Britain undoubtedly failed to fully utilise its peacemaking potential in Cyprus between July 1974 and 1980, its inaction does not make it a guilty party. It acted within the bounds of its perceptions, interests and obligations and one would be hard-pressed to prove that it actually failed in its role as a guarantor power.

Greece. Greece's attitude towards peacemaking in Cyprus in the July 1974-80 period was in marked contrast to that of the Greek military which had ruled Greece from 1967 to July 1974. There was no desire now to dictate policy to Cyprus, and the Greek government no longer saw the Cyprus issue as a paramount concern. Nor did it have the means to persuade the key players to adopt a more favourable position towards the Greek Cypriots.

The position of Greece in relation to the events of July 1974 is central, particularly as it was a Greek-staged coup that led to the Turkish invasion. However, its role was diminished after the collapse of the Junta on 22 July 1974 and the restoration of democracy. In the preceding months the regime had been led by Ioannides, formerly commander of the military police, who ousted Papadopoulos in November 1973. Cyprus was an issue from which Ioannides could potentially gain some domestic political capital, but not as long as Makarios remained in charge there.

The regime's unpopularity was a major factor in its decision to stage a coup in Cyprus. As one writer has observed, it was 'a desperate attempt by the Ioannides Junta to consolidate its precarious position by gaining popular support through a nationalist triumph'[93] in the belief, as another commentator has remarked, that it 'would crown its rule with glory and legitimise its continued existence'.[94]

Crucially, the Colonels acted in the belief that Turkey would not react, possibly following assurances from Turkey itself[95] and from the United States[96] to that effect. But even if this had been the case, their incredible act in appointing Sampson, who was well known for his dislike of the Turks, as the new president effectively ruined any chance of success, and gave the Turks, in the words of a senior Turkish official, 'the opportunity to solve our problems once and for all'.[97]

However, the first unexpected outcome of the coup was Makarios's safe escape, which provoked this reported telephone exchange between the conspirators:

> *Ioannides*: 'I see the old — has escaped. Where could he be now?'
> *Sampson*: 'On the mountains, heading for Kykkos [the monastery]. I hope to have him arrested within two or three hours.'
> *Ioannides*: 'Nicky, I want his head. You shall bring it to me yourself, OK, Nicky?'[98]

On 21 July 1974, the day after the Turkish invasion, Ioannides decided to go to war with Turkey, which caused the immediate collapse both of the Junta and its puppet regime in Nicosia. Constantive Karamanlis was asked to return from exile and form a civilian government. On 24 July he was sworn in as the new prime minister.

The first important decision of Karamanlis's government over Cyprus was to give public backing to Makarios as its head of state[99] despite his absence from the island at the time. Its second decision was not to go to war with Turkey after the second Turkish invasion of Cyprus. This was later followed by Greece's withdrawal from NATO, on the grounds that the alliance had demonstrated pro-Turkish bias over Cyprus and had failed to help the Greek people. This was in fact an act of great statesmanship by Karamanlis. Callaghan described the events after the second Turkish invasion as follows:

> At 5.00 a.m. on the same morning the Greek Cabinet met in the Ministry of Defence. With the exception of the Prime Minister, Constantine Karamanlis, those who were present demanded that Greece declare war on Turkey forthwith. The Prime Minister...proposed an alternative that Greece should request NATO's immediate assistance in accordance with the dictum that an attack on one is an attack on all. [...] He withdrew Greece from NATO and, unwelcome though

> that was, by doing so he saved his country from a war that would have been disastrous for the future of the new democracy.[100]

However, refusing to retaliate against Turkey had a negative psychological impact on the Greek Cypriots as it was an admission by the Greeks, for the first time in the modern history of Cyprus, that the old Ottoman enemy had the upper hand and they were unable to do anything about it. It also demonstrated that Greek and Greek Cypriot interests were not necessarily the same or even compatible. In Karamanlis's view, the Cyprus issue could not be allowed to interfere with Greece's foreign policy aims such as securing membership of the EEC.[101] As he himself explained in a speech in August 1974,

> Armed opposition to the Turks in Cyprus was made impossible by reason of distance and also by reason of the accomplished facts. [...] And it could not be attempted without the risk of weakening the defence of Greece itself. At this point I wish to declare categorically that the defence capability of Greece is absolute throughout the land.[102]

So in direct opposition to Turkey, which dominated the main outlines of Turkish Cypriot policies and saw its interest as inextricably intertwined with the fate of Cyprus, Karamanlis began a new chapter of separation between Greece and Cyprus. His vulnerable position as a democratic leader during a time of high tension with Turkey might have prompted a general hardening of Greece's position but, on the contrary, Karamanlis started a dialogue with Turkey. A clear manifestation of the rapprochment occurred on 31 May 1975 when the two premiers, Karamanlis and Demirel, met in Brussels and pledged to settle the Cyprus problem by peaceful means. That meeting eventually led on 12 December to an agreement between their foreign ministers in Brussels during a NATO summit. The agreement, known as the Brussels Accord, contained the following points:[103]

(1) The Secretary-General of the United Nations to be asked to appeal to the representatives of the two communities to continue their talks without prior conditions, with a view to arriving at a package deal on an agenda containing the following subjects: territorial issues, federal structure, powers of central government.
(2) Details of these subjects to be examined by two subcommittees to the extent that would be required.
(3) The two ministers to encourage the representatives of the two communities to respond positively to the appeal of the Secretary-General and accept the earliest possible date for the first meeting under his chairmanship.
(4) Until the talks were completed all the parties concerned to avoid revealing the content of the points on which there might be provisional agreement since that would be contrary to the principle of a package agreement. The parties would also abstain from statements which could jeopardise the progress already made. Therefore each party reserved the right to deny statements of leakages

which could be contrary to the present agreement.
(5) The Ministers to meet from time to time to survey the progress made and if necessary, to deal with difficulties arising; and
(6) to examine all problems affecting relations between the two countries.

However, the Brussels Accord, significant though it was, failed to produce any result, since it was too general and failed to address any of the particular and controversial issues, such as the three basic freedoms. It was also weakened by lack of representation by the two Cypriot communities.

Karamanlis's soft approach towards the Cyprus problem continued up to the end of his premiership in 1980 when he was succeeded by George Rallis. In October 1980 Greece re-entered NATO, thus putting an end to its official protest over the Turkish invasion of Cyprus, which had remained in force till that time. This move typified the relatively relaxed policy of avoiding war with Turkey and continuing to support the intercommunal talks. Greek/Greek Cypriot relations during this period were cordial, as Cyprus received large sums in aid from Greece and Greek Cypriot politicians paid regular visits there. This period marked the end of Greece's desire to sacrifice its interest for the sake of Hellenistic ideas incompatible with political realities and showed that Greek and Greek Cypriot interests were not always the same despite the ethnic links between the two peoples. Overall, Greece's attitude was supportive of peacemaking in Cyprus during this period.

Turkey. Turkey's attitude towards Cyprus in this period was crucial, since it alone was in a position to change the negative stance of the Turkish Cypriot leadership. However, despite its public support for the peace process, it failed to use its influence on Denktash to persuade him to implement the 1977 and 1979 High-Level Agreements.

After the events of July 1974 Turkey's attitude to the Cyprus problem became the decisive one, so that any solution which did not have Turkey's blessing was inconceivable. While its involvement in Cyprus in the pre-July 1974 period was a reaction to developments, the period since then has seen it as the key actor. Its troops in the north of the island and its strong influence over the Turkish Cypriot leadership have been the two main factors for Turkey's pivotal role in the Cyprus problem after July 1974. Its policy in the period derived, as before, from two principles: its security interests and the wellbeing of the Turkish Cypriots, both of which had been threatened by the coup of 1974. By examing the motives behind Turkey's invasion it is possible to understand its position on peacemaking in Cyprus in the years that followed.[104]

Turkey's inclination to strike for success by military means was strengthened by public opinion, which thirsted for a decisive move against the old Greek enemy, as illustrated by the then Turkish naval commander, Admiral Karacan, who remarked to the premier Bulent Ecevit, after the coup: 'if we turn back from Cyprus as before I won't be able to remain naval commander-in-chief and you won't be able to remain prime minister.[105] Unlike Inönü in 1964 and Demirel in 1967, Ecevit himself was in favour of a strong response. Because Turkish efforts to involve Britain in its military operation against Cyprus failed to produce any result, last-minute military preparations were conducted to launch the invasion. Later, at the Geneva talks, it became clear that Turkey was in no mood to negotiate and if its proposals on Cyprus were rejected, it would use its military machine again, which is exactly what happened.[106]

A second motive for the invasion was the fact that the coup in Cyprus had brought the possibility of *Enosis* closer to reality, and in the eyes of the Turkish policy-makers, other considerations apart, this would have been detrimental to Turkish security interests; Greece could not be allowed to dominate this area of the Mediterranean.[107] There was also a suspicion among Turkish officials that the United States government was about to recognise the new puppet regime in Nicosia,[108] which would have posed further danger to Turkish security interests.

The third reason for the invasion was to protect the lives of Turkish Cypriots. At a news conference on 14 August 1974, Ecevit stated that the objective of the military operation in Cyprus was 'to put an end to the suffering the Turkish Cypriots have had to endure over the years'.[109] However, there is doubt whether this could have been the prime reason for the decision to invade: the coup had in no way endangered the lives of Turkish Cypriots. It was the second Turkish military invasion on 14 August which provoked hostilities against the Turkish Cypriots by the Greek Cypriots. Before this, the situation in the island had been more or less quiet.[110] In any case, the invasion went far beyond what would have been required to protect the Turkish Cypriots.[111]

Lastly, Turkey saw military action as a golden opportunity to make a decisively advantageous move against the Greeks. It could not now be deterred by the United States or the threat of Soviet military intervention. As one Turkish diplomat put it, 'Unlike 1964 and 1967 the United States leverage on us in 1974 was minimal. We could no longer be scared off by threats that the Soviet Union would intercede.'[112] Again, unlike 1964 and 1967, Turkey was now militarily fully equipped for a landing,[113] increasing still further the appeal of a military operation against Cyprus.

The Turkish invasion transformed the problem of Cyprus in a number of ways. First, it changed from a problem of intercommunal strife to one of foreign occupation, which in the eyes of the international community made Turkey the real culprit. Further, it confirmed that on the Turkish side it was Turkey that was making the decisive moves in

Cyprus. This had important implications for peacemaking, since it was now clearly Turkey and not the Turkish Cypriots who had to be persuaded to accept a settlement.

Secondly, the Turkish invasion turned the Greek Cypriots into the bereaved party in the Cyprus conflict. Having already enjoyed the support of the international community, their victimisation at the hands of the powerful Turkish military gave the sympathy of the international community, which they enjoyed, a new emotional dimension. A trend developed thereafter whereby efforts were made by each community to convince the world that it was the aggrieved party in the conflict; hence the huge propaganda war that has been going on ever since. This was and has continued to be a negative development for peacemaking in Cyprus in two ways: first, the propaganda war has fuelled past enmities and prevented an intercommunal rapproachement, and secondly, each community felt that the further ahead it could get in this intercommunal cold war, the more chance it had of obtaining concessions from the other side in any settlement. Winning the propaganda war became an end in itself, in direct opposition to peacemaking objectives in Cyprus. Thirdly, the invasion automatically linked the Cyprus problem to a range of conflicting issues between Turkey and Greece effectively making Cyprus a bargaining chip for Turkey; according to one report, the second phase of the Turkish invasion was carried out specifically for this reason.[114] Naturally such attitudes took, and continue to take, the problem of Cyprus out of context, and in a way negate all peacemaking efforts towards a settlement. Fourthly, the Turkish invasion of Cyprus was a flagrant violation of the UN charter and the Security Council resolutions, and so reduced the credibility of the UN and UNFICYP, which took some forty casualties in the fighting, seven of them fatal. The invasion also showed us the vulnerability of any peacekeeping initiative that lacks a viable peacemaking mechanism. Finally, the invasion now ensured that any solution would be based on federation rather than a unitary state since it forced the acquiescence of the Greek Cypriots. However, although the acceptance by them of federation as the basis of negotiations aroused hope among observers, it did not lead to a settlement.

Turkey's attitude towards the Cyprus problem in this period was also largely affected by its internal politics. Bulent Ecevit's government, which authorised the invasion, was itself a coalition and thus had to take into account the views of its partner in power. However, the coalition collapsed in November 1974 when Ecevit was opposed by Erbakan, his coalition partner and deputy, who rejected an offer of talks over Cyprus with the US Secretary of State Henry Kissinger. Between 1973 and 1979 there were seven governments in Turkey, only four of which had a majority in the National Assembly, making it difficult to take unpopular decisions that risked upsetting the minority parties. When the army took power in Turkey in September 1980, many hoped that strong government immune to party politics could perhaps open the way to a settlement.

The impact of Turkish domestic politics on the Turkish Cypriots was direct, noticeable and negative in its effect on peacemaking between July 1974 and 1980. One example is the Turkish parliamentary elections of 1977, which effectively blocked the Turkish Cypriots' proposals in the intercommunal talks for three months pending the outcome.[115] Also, Turkey's financial support for the Turkish Cypriots – reaching $10,143,750 in 1980[116] – tended to integrate the Turkish Cypriot economy with the Turkish economy, thus increasing the dependence of the minority community in Cyprus on its mother-country and reducing its freedom to cooperate in the peacemaking process.

Internationally Turkey was condemned after its invasion of Cyprus. Consecutive UN resolutions, the Non-Aligned movement and the Commonwealth all demanded withdrawal of foreign troops from Cyprus. However, this never went further than words. The only action taken against Turkey was by the United States government, under pressure from Congress, which resulted in an embargo on grants, credits and commercial military sales. In retaliation the Turkish government took over most of the United States bases and closed down its monitoring stations in Turkey. In general, international pressure on Turkey took only a moral form and failed to persuade it to take positive steps towards a settlement. The main reason for the West's unwillingness to press Turkey over Cyprus was its strategic significance – not merely important, but as the British foreign secretary Lord Carrington put it, 'essential'.[117]

Yet there were important considerations which would have made a peaceful solution in Cyprus useful for Turkey. First and foremost, it would have enhanced Turkey's international prestige, and hence its image in the Third World, where there was almost universal support for the Greek Cypriots. It would have helped Greco-Turkish relations, already boosted by the Brussels Accord. Economically, too, the Turkish Cypriots had proved a burden for Turkey, which was already performing rather poorly. And finally, the security interests of Turkey would have been better served by a stable and secure Cyprus. In the long run, some argued, Turkey would come to regret its occupation of Cyprus. As James Callaghan remarked in the aftermath of the invasion, 'Today the Republic of Cyprus is the prisoner of the Turkish army. Tomorrow the Turkish army will find that it will become the prisoner of the Republic of Cyprus.'[118]

However, in the eyes of Turkish policy-makers, the July 1974-80 period was a successful one where Cyprus was concerned. Turkey's military presence in the island had secured the interests of Turkey and the lives of Turkish Cypriots, at least for the immediate future. It had managed to assert effective military control over a third of the island without provoking any far-reaching international reaction beyond verbal condemnation and was not prepared to forgo such an advantageous position for a settlement that did not take full account of its strategic interests.

The United States. Between July 1974 and 1980 the United States took a relaxed attitude towards peacemaking in Cyprus. Save for the immediate threat of a Greco-Turkish war in July and August 1974, the democratic government in Greece had shown that it would not go to war with Turkey over Cyprus, thus greatly reducing US anxieties over the Cyprus problem. The 1978 American-British-Canadian Plan, already explained, was the pinnacle of US peacemaking efforts in Cyprus in this period.

US policy on Cyprus in the July 1974-80 period continued, as in the proceeding years, to be chiefly governed by concern over Soviet influence in the region and particularly by the need to avoid an extension of that influence in the Middle East.[119] Another important concern was the intra-alliance cohesion of NATO; it was essential that Cyprus should not be allowed to drive Greece and Turkey, both members of NATO, into a war with each other. For US policy-makers the best way of avoiding this would be the removal of Makarios from office or at least a reduction of his authority on the island. The prevailing view was that he was 'unreliable, demagogic, anti-western, and obstructive to any final settlement of the Cyprus problem'.[120] The 'Castro of the Mediterranean', as he was known in some circles in Washington, had proved a liability to US interests; as Kissinger put it to a Greek Cypriot official with magnificent tact, 'We think of your president as a man who is much too big for so small an island.'[121]

In the context of the Cold War, Turkey was seen to be a more important country than Greece. In 1974 Kissinger had made a cold-blooded strategic decision that Turkey was more important to US security and to NATO than Greece, with its new and unpredictable government and volatile electorate.[122] As one US official remarked, 'Let's say that Greece is Denmark and Turkey is Germany. We may be fonder of the Danes, but we need the Germans more.'[123]

Since the Greek-staged coup seemed to fulfill the US policy objectives of dealing with the 'Makarios factor' and tilting towards Turkey, some observers saw the US government as being in favour of the coup,[124] pointing to its failure to join in the universal condemnation[125] and to the US veto of the Security Council draft resolution condemning Greece for the role it had played.[126] In the light of the desire of the United States to see Makarios removed, this position is understandable; the guarded NATO statement on the Turkish invasion, which in one observer's view was so restrained it could 'amount almost to approval',[127] was also unsurprising, given Turkey's strategic significance. Kissinger's private confession that he was not prepared to stop the Turks until they had achieved their territorial objective[128] confirmed the way the United States saw its priorities.

The US government's attitude aroused bitter feelings among Greeks and Greek Cypriots alike. Some 20,000 Greek Americans demonstrated in front of the White House, and similar demonstrations took place in Athens and Nicosia. On 19 August 1974 the US ambassador in Cyprus, Roger P. Davies, was assassinated there. At the time of these events the Nixon administration was embroiled in the Watergate scandal, which led eventually to the President's resignation. Other pressing international issues also demanded Kissinger's attention, making Cyprus 'a far-off blip on [his] storm charts'.[129]

The Ford administration modified US policy by deploring the Turkish invasion, and under pressure from Congress it imposed an embargo against Turkey on 5 February 1975. The coming to office of President Carter in 1977 initially raised hopes as he announced a new initiative and appointed a former Secretary of State, Clark Clifford, to look into the Cyprus problem;[130] however, nothing came of this. In November 1978 the joint American-British-Canadian Plan already referred to was drafted and put to the disputing parties but was rejected by the Cyprus government. The Plan was the high-point of United States efforts in this period to solve the Cyprus problem peacefully.

The Cold War and the policy of containment, together with the importance of intra-alliance cohesion in NATO, dominated US policy and restricted its peacemaking ability in Cyprus during this period. Although the United States might have used its considerable influence in Greece and Turkey,[131] and could possibly have precluded the events of July and August 1974, it decided instead on a policy of 'constructive ambiguity',[132] continuing to support the presence of UNFICYP as minimising the likelihood of another armed conflict in Cyprus that might lead to a Greco-Turkish war. By 1980 Greece was back in NATO and the embargo against Turkey had been lifted. For the United States the worst – a Greco-Turkish war – had been averted but a solution, as in the past, had continued to eluded it.

The Soviet Union. Soviet policy over Cyprus from the coup and the invasion to 1980 derived as before from two principles: to maintain the independence and non-alignment of Cyprus and at the same time try to bring about a rift within the south-eastern flank of NATO. The events of July and August 1974 presented the Soviets with an opportunity to internationalise the Cyprus problem further, and also to disrupt the Atlantic Alliance. However, in practice they had little success with either objective. Their peacemaking ability in Cyprus, save for their political approval of UNFICYP, remained rather limited during the July 1974-80 period.

Support for independence and non-alignment was a form of support for Makarios, since the Archbishop, much to the Soviets' approval, was a staunch believer in both these principles. Makarios's departure from Cyprus in the aftermath of the coup – brief as it turned out to be – was received with dismay in the Soviet Union, which is why it offered to help Turkey reinstate him.[133] It was also worried about Turkey's partitionist intentions in Cyprus, leading Soviet policy-makers in 1974 to seek improved relations with Greece, which at the time was manifesting anti-American sentiments.[134] Soviet policy was indicated only a few days after the proclamation of the 'Turkish Federated State of Cyprus' when in a joint communiqué issued by the British prime minister Harold Wilson and the Soviet leader Leonid Brezhnev on 17 February 1975 in Moscow, both countries stated that they would only recognise 'the one lawful government of Cyprus headed by President Makarios'.[135] To further its courtship of Turkey and make trouble for NATO it held up the Security Council Resolution calling for a ceasefire in the immediate aftermath of the Turkish invasion.[136] In fact, the Soviet Union's attitude was highly satisfactory for the Turkish government: Ecevit remarked after the fighting: 'Not only the United States, but the Soviet Union tried to be objective and constructive *vis-à-vis* the recent eruptions and we don't have anything to complain about regarding the attitude of the two countries.'[137]

The Soviet Union's most direct attempt at peacemaking took place on 24 August 1974 when it suggested an international conference on the Cyprus problem, which would have further internationalised it and given the Soviets a say in any solution. Turkey rejected the idea, however,[138] and nothing came of it.

As with the United States, Soviet policy on Cyprus continued to be influenced by the Cold War: continued support for AKEL, periodic sanctioning of UNFICYP in the Security Council, support for President Makarios, attempts to establish some sort of rapport with Turkey, and moves to convene an international conference – all derived from the two main objectives of maintaining the independence and the non-alignment of Cyprus and trying to disrupt NATO. In the light of these objectives, which ran counter to those of the United States, the Soviet Union lacked the potential to contribute significantly to peacemaking in Cyprus in the July 1974-80 period. However, its support for UNFICYP was noteworthy.

The United Nations. The United Nations remained the main intermediary agency with the potential to bring about a peaceful settlement to the

Cyprus problem. The good offices of the Secretary-General were employed to this end, and the Vienna talks, as well as the High-Level Agreements of 1977 and 1979, were all conducted under UN auspices. In general its role was positive, but it could only operate within the framework provided by member states, particularly the Security Council. However, UNFICYP continued its peacekeeping function in the island during this period.

The 1974 coup and the subsequent Turkish invasion of Cyprus affected UN peacemaking in a number of ways. First of all, these events destroyed all previous UN peacemaking efforts, which had been going on in the form of the 1968-July 1974 intercommunal talks. As the problem was transformed from one of intercommunal strife to one of foreign occupation, a new basis for negotiations between the disputants had to be established. This meant a radical change in the nature of the objectives to be sought as, for instance, the 'unitary state' objective was replaced by 'federation', rendering fruitless the 1968-74 Intercommunal Talks.[139] Secondly, the Turkish invasion undermined the credibility of the UN globally, and particularly in Cyprus. The casualties sustained by UNFICYP during the invasion highlighted the weakest point of its mandate, namely its inability to use arms other than in self-defence, which made it no deterrent to the Turkish army. Despite Secretary-General Waldheim's suggestion to extend the mandate of the force to enable it to resist the second Turkish invasion,[140] UNFICYP was prepared to withdraw in the face of a Turkish advance,[141] although in the event it fought valiantly for the defence of Nicosia's international airport.

Nevertheless, the consequent diminished degree of confidence in the UN was naturally a setback for its peacemaking efforts in Cyprus. These were twofold: one was the adoption of various resolutions by the Security Council and the General Assembly and the other was support from the Secretary-General for the intercommunal talks. From July 1974 to June 1980, there were twenty-four Security Council and six General Assembly resolutions on the Cyprus problem, all supporting the independence, sovereignty and territorial integrity of Cyprus and calling for meaningful negotiations between all the disputants. In fact, it was in response to paragraph 5 of Resolution 353 of the Security Council of 20 July 1974 that the guarantor powers entered into Geneva talks.

The moral authority of these resolutions was a constant irritant to Turkey and Turkish Cypriots. Turkey often had to face the embarrassment of being in an extreme minority over the Cyprus issue among all the other nations of the world in the General Assembly, which proved so uncomfortable that on 1 November 1974 it voted with other members of the Assembly for Resolution 3212 (XXIX) which urged 'the speedy withdrawal of all foreign armed forces and foreign military presence and personnel from the Republic of Cyprus'.

One significant development in the resolutions after July 1974 was their recommendation that intercommunal talks should take place on an 'equal footing'. This phrase was first used in Resolution 3212 (XXIX) of 1 November 1974 and was positive in officially recognising the equal status of the Turkish Cypriots as citizens of the Republic of Cyprus. And in Security Council Resolution 367 of 12 March 1975, for the first time since the 1967 crisis, the Secretary-General was asked to attempt a new settlement, indicating a belief that he could perhaps achieve better results if he were given sufficient backing. Throughout the July 1974-1980 period the Secretary-General made repeated efforts to get the intercommunal talks underway, arranging the ceasefire on 22 July 1974 and organising meetings with the parties concerned;[142] Security Council Resolution 361 of 30 August 1974 specifically applauded these efforts. Following the Brussels Accord between Greece and Turkey, the Secretary-General seized the initiative by inviting the representatives of the two communities to Vienna for further talks. His role and that of his special representative in Cyprus in arranging the Makarios- Denktash meeting of 1977[143] and the Kyprianou-Denktash meeting of 1979[144] were also significant. Intercommunal talks were an important way for the two Cypriot communities to exchange views frankly and for some, including the Secretary-General himself, the only way of achieving a settlement.[145]

The UN's involvement in the Cyprus dispute led to considerable humanitarian work in the aftermath of the Turkish invasion, which produced thousands of refugees and many missing persons. UNFICYP also played an invaluable part in easing tension[146] and establishing a semblance of normality; this was important for peacemaking, which is all but impossible when the disputants are involved in physical combat.

The question is why, despite all these efforts, the UN failed to settle the Cyprus problem between July 1974 and 1980. As before, differences with the US persisted,[147] depriving it of the backing of its most powerful member. Secondly, the UN continued to lack the mandate, and the political and military power, to implement its resolutions. This weakness was highlighted by the former Cypriot president Kyprianou, who on 6 October 1977 urged the General Assembly 'to impress upon the Security Council the necessity of taking all measures warranted by the situation in order to bring about the long overdue implementation of the Council's resolutions on Cyprus'.[148] The General Assembly eventually responded with a request to the Security Council (Resolution 33/15 of 9 November 1978) to 'examine the question of the implementation, within a time-frame of its relevant resolutions and consider and adopt thereafter, if necessary, all appropriate and practical measures under the Charter of the United Nations for ensuring the implementation of the resolution of the United Nations on Cyprus.' However, this appeal, though repeated in its subsequent resolutions on Cyprus, did not lead to any development.

The general lack of confidence in the UN at the time was also damaging. Its failure to draft a resolution immediately condemning the coup in Cyprus had understandably disappointed Cypriots and non-Cypriots alike. The Soviet Union, which had been a staunch defender of Cyprus's territorial integrity before 1974, was now content merely to give verbal support for the UN's unimplemented resolutions.

Finally, the United Nations does not possess magical properties: anything which it is to do that requires more than the voluntary contribution of the disputants depends on key UN members putting the right sort of pressure on them, which in this case simply did not happen. However, in spite of its failure to conclude a settlement, the UN was helpful in a number of ways. Its resolutions acted as constant reminders to the international community of the need to resolve the Cyprus problem, and by recognising the Cyprus government despite protests from Turkey it upheld the Charter's principles concerning the illegality of occupation of foreign territory. The regret it expressed (Security Council Resolution 367 of 12 March 1975) over the proclaimed Turkish Federated State in the occupied north of Cyprus reflected this principle, while its humanitarian work in housing refugees and seeking information about missing persons was also commendable.

The events of July and August 1974 proved that with so little authority the UN cannot be what the world community expects it to be. This is true in peacekeeping as well as in peacemaking. As a report of a study mission said:

> The effectiveness of UNFICYP's role on Cyprus was shattered with the invasion of the Turkish army. The mandate of UNFICYP under these conditions made it a 'peacekeeping force' in name only. As it watched [the] Turkish army move across Cyprus, UNFICYP became more of a 'peace observing force', watching the breakdown of peace, with no power to maintain it, much less to enforce it.[149]

Yet although the UN's peacemaking in the July 1974-80 period in Cyprus proved unsuccessful, it did its best within the parameters set by the international community for a peaceful settlement.

Following the Turkish invasion, the Cyprus problem changed dramatically. With huge numbers of troops in the northern part of the island, Turkey became the key outside power. The question of a foreign army occupying territory of the Cyprus Republic was now added to intercommunal mistrust, which greatly intensified after July and August 1974. The net result was that Turkey's blessing was a necessary condition if any settlement was to have a chance of success. However, Turkey was in no hurry to come to any agreement over Cyprus, and there was not sufficient pressure on it from the West, particularly from the United States, to make it more flexible on the issue. Accordingly, the Turkish Cypriots considerably toughened their stance in negotiations with the Greek Cypriots.

The Geneva talks, the Vienna talks (conducted under UN auspices) and the American-British-Canadian initiative were the three peacemaking efforts, of which the only tangible results were the 1977 and the 1979 High-Level Agreements between the two community leaders, which in practice achieved nothing. Although the attitudes of Turkey and the Turkish Cypriots were largely responsible for the lack of progress in peacemaking, it was the Greek Cypriots who rejected the American-British-Canadian Initiative of November 1978, although hitherto they had been the more conciliatory side.

NOTES

1. Quoted by Laurence Stern, 'Bitter Lessons: How we failed in Cyprus', *Foreign Policy*, no. 19, summer 1975, p. 53.
2. *Ibid.*
3. *Ibid.*, p. 54; see also Christopher Hitchens, *Cyprus*, London: Quartet, 1984, pp. 81 and 82.
4. Polyvios G. Poliviou, *Cyprus: Conflict and Negotiation 1960-1980*, London: Duckworth, 1980, p. 154.
5. *Keesing's 20* (12-18 August 1974): 26605.
6. *UN Doc.* S/11398, 30 July 1974, paras 2 and 3.
7. James Callaghan, *Time and Chance*, London: Collins, 1987, p. 349.
8. *Cyprus 1974: Hearings before the Committee on Foreign Affairs*, London: HMSO, 1974, p. 5.
9. *UN Doc.* S/11433, 10 August 1974, para. 8.
10. Glafkos Clerides *Cyprus: My Deposition*, Nicosia: Alithia Publishing, vol. 4, 1992, pp. 49, 51, 53.
11. *A Study Mission Report*, 93rd Cong., 2nd Sess. p. 16.
12. Callaghan, op. cit., p. 355.
13. L. Stern, *The Wrong Horse: The Politics of Intervention and the Failure of American Diplomacy*, New York: Times Books, 1978, p. 133.
14. Clerides, vol. 4, op. cit., p. 259.
15. *UN Doc.* S/11717, 9 June 1975, para. 66.
16. *Ibid.*, para. 53.
17. *Ibid.*, para. 66.
18. Clerides, vol. 4, op. cit., p. 330.
19. For the full text of the proposals of the two sides see *UN Doc.* S/12093, 5 June 1976, Annex I and Annex II.
20. *UN Doc.* S/12323, 30 April 1977, para. 5.
21. For the full text of the Greek Cypriot and Turkish Cypriot proposals see ibid., paras. 7, 9-13, annex II, III, IV, V.
22. *UN Doc.* S/13369, 31 May 1979.

23. Pamphlet published by the Press and Information Office of the Cyprus government in October 1979; see also the *New York Times*, 29 November 1978.
24. Michael Attalides, *Cyprus: Nationalism and International Politics*, Edinburgh: Q Press, 1979, p. 162.
25. Nicola Mandic, 'Cyprus After Makarios', *Review of International Affairs*, vol. XXVIII, 660, 5 October 1977, p. 26.
26. *New York Times*, 7 November 1974, p. 18a.
27. Zenon Stavrinides, *The Cyprus Conflict: National Identity and Statehood*, Nicosia: Loris Stavrinides Press, p. 92.
28. *UN Doc.* S/11789, 5 August 1975.
29. *UN Doc.* S/11900, 8 December 1975.
30. *UN Doc.* S/14778, 1 December 1980.
31. *Newsweek*, 16 December 1974, p. 46.
32. See in this regard a chapter by Dimitri Kitsikis, in T.A. Coulombis and S.M. Hicks (eds), *United States Foreign Policy Towards Greece and Cyprus: The Clash of Principle and Pragmatism*, Washington, DC: Centre for Mediterranean Studies and American Hellenic Institute, 1975.
33. *Philelephtheros*, 6 August 1977, p. 1 (translation by Maria Mirbagheri).
34. *Financial Times*, 24 July 1974.
35. Ibid.
36. Pierre Oberling, *The Road to Bellapais*, New York: Social Science Monographs, Boulder, 1982, p. 197.
37. Ibid.
38. *New York Times*, 7 November 1974, p. 18a.
39. Ibid.
40. George, S. Kaloudis, *The Role of the UN in Cyprus from 1964 to 1979*, unpublished Ph.D. thesis, University of Kansas, 1982, p. 113.
41. For an elaborate account of the Greek-Cypriot position see *Cyprus Intercommunal Talks, Following the Turkish Invasion of July-August 1974*, Nicosia: Cyprus Govt. Press and Information Office, April 1982, pp. 42-6.
42. *Dagbladet*, 12 March 1977, quoted by Oberling, op. cit., p. 207.
43. Mandic, op. cit., p. 26.
44. Oberling, op. cit., p. 210.
45. *The Economist*, 31 May 1979.
46. *Hurriet*, 5 March 1980, p. 58 (translation by Reza Dehghan).
47. *Cyprus Mail*, 13 November 1980, p. 1.
48. Stavrinides, op. cit., p. 96.
49. Ibid.
50. *Turkish Demographic Manipulations in Cyprus*, Nicosia, June 1987, p. 8.
51. *Turkish Press on Cyprus*, Nicosia: Cyprus Govt. Press and Information Office, 1980, p. 32.
52. *The Economist*, 19 November 1975, p. 56.
53. *Turkish Press on Cyprus*, p. 33.
54. Callaghan, op. cit., 354.
55. *The Economist*, 20 July 1974, Survey Section, p. 18.
56. *Turkish Press on Cyprus*, p. 58.
57. Polyviou, *Cyprus: Conflict*, p. 164.
58. Ertekun, Necati, *The Cyprus Dispute and the Birth of the Turkish Republic of Northern Cyprus*, Nicosia: K. Rustem and Bro., 2nd edn, 1984, p. 31.
59. Polyviou, *Cyprus: Conflict*, p. 164.
60. *UN Doc.* S/11624, 18 February 1975, Annex B.
61. Ibid.
62. Mandic, op. cit., p. 26.
63. Oberling, op. cit., p. 179.

64. Stavrinides, op. cit., p. 90.
65. Callaghan, op. cit., pp. 353-4.
66. *UN Doc.* S/12723, 31 May 1978, para. 52.
67. *UN Doc.* S/11900, 8 December 1975, paras. 52, 53, 55.
68. Nancy Crawshaw, 'Cyprus after Makarios: Prospects for a Settlement', *The World Today*, vol. 34, no. 1, January 1978, p. 32.
69. Stephen Ryan, 'Ethnic Conflict and the International System: Foreign Involvement in the Cyprus Problem 1974-1982', unpubl. Ph.D. thesis, London School of Economics, 1984, p. 181.
70. Crawshaw, op. cit., p. 35.
71. Oberling, op. cit., p. 225.
72. Ibid.
73. Ibid.
74. *UN Doc.* A/33/113, 26 May 1978.
75. *The Guardian*, 3 November 1979.
76. For the texts of some of the resolutions by Conferences of Foreign Ministers of Islamic States, see *UN Doc.* S/12085, 26 May 1985, A/32/133, 7 July 1977.
77. *UN Doc.* A/33/233, 12 September 1978.
78. Ryan, op. cit., p. 205.
79. Kaloudis, op. cit., p. 113.
80. Ryan, op. cit., p. 250.
81. Callaghan, op. cit., p. 353.
82. Ryan, op. cit., p. 244.
83. Callaghan, op. cit., p. 341.
84. Polyviou, *Cyprus: Conflict*, p. 162.
85. Callaghan, op. cit., p. 342.
86. Report of the Select Committee on Cyprus, Parliamentary Papers, vol. 17, 1975-6, p. 763X, para. 22.
87. Polyviou, *Cyprus: Conflict*, p. 157.
88. Parliamentary Debates, 5th series, vol. 911, 19 May 1976, col. 1400.
89. Callaghan, op. cit., p. 357.
90. Parliamentary Debates, 5th series, vol. 891, 30 April 1975, col. 453.
91. Parliamentary Debates, 5th series, vol. 977, 22 January 1980, cols 147-8.
92. Parliamentary Debates, 5th Series, vol. 958, 20 November 1978, col. 448.
93. Mouzelis, N.P., *Modern Greece: Facets of Underdevelopment*, London: Macmillan, 1978, p. 130.
94. See Oberling, op. cit., p. 153.
95. Stern, *Bitter*, op. cit., p. 56.
96. Attalides, *Cyprus: Nationalism*, p. 170.
97. Stern, *Bitter*, p. 63.
98. Hitchens, op. cit., pp. 93-4.
99. *The Economist*, 27 February 1974, p. 16.
100. Callaghan, op. cit., p. 355-6.
101. For elaboration on this point see Van Coufoudakis, 'Defining Greek Foreign Policy Objectives' in Howard R. Penniman, (ed.), *Greece at the Polls: The National Elections of 1974 and 1977*, Washington, DC: American Enterprise Institute for Public Policy Research, 1981.
102. *Keesings*, 1974, p. 26710.
103. Ertekun, *The Cyprus Dispute*, op. cit., Appendix 32, p. 273.
104. See Sharon Anderholm Weiner, *Turkish Foreign Policy Decision Making on the Cyprus Issue: A Comparative Analysis of Three Crises*, unpubl. Ph.D. thesis, Duke University, 1980, p. 306.
105. Hitchens, op. cit., p. 96.

106. For an elaborate account of the Turkish Invasion of Cyprus see M.A. Birand, *30 Hot Days*, Nicosia: K. Rustem and Bro. 1985.
107. Ibid., p. 3.
108. Stern, *The Wrong*, op. cit., pp. 113-115.
109. *New York Times*, 15 August 1974, p. 15d.
110. UN Doc. S/11353, Add. 20, 12 August 1974, para. 1.
111. Ryan, op. cit., p. 211.
112. Stern, *The Wrong*, op. cit., p. 63.
113. Attalides, *Cyprus: Nationalism*, p. 174.
114. North Atlantic Assembly, 'Report on the Activities of the Subcommittee on the Southern Flank', September 1975, quoted in Attalides, *Cyprus: Nationalism*, p. 177, note 77.
115. William, see Hale, 'Turkey's Inconclusive Election', *The World Today*, vol. 33, no. 7, July 1977.
116. Oberling, op. cit., p. 225.
117. *The Guardian*, 10 November 1980.
118. *UN Doc.*, S/PV 1973, 19 November 1976, para. 75.
119. Callaghan, op. cit., p. 339.
120. Stern, *Bitter*, p. 58.
121. Ibid., p. 57.
122. Ibid., p. 74.
123. Ibid., p. 75.
124. Attalides, *Cyprus: Nationalism*, p. 168.
125. Polyviou, *Cyprus: Conflict*, p. 156.
126. Birand, op. cit., p. 14.
127. Ibid., p. 27.
128. Stern, *Bitter*, op. cit., p. 73.
129. Ibid., p. 27.
130. Crawshaw, op. cit., p. 31.
131. Callaghan, op. cit., p. 341.
132. Oberling, op. cit., p. 162.
133. Attalides, *Cyprus: Nationalism*, p. 162.
134. Oberling, op. cit., p. 184.
135. *UN Doc.* S/11659, 21 March 1975.
136. 'Gemeinsamkeiten and Unterschiede in der Haltung Moskaus and Pekings zum Zypern-Konflikt', *Frankfurter Allgemeine Zeitung*, 24 July 1974, quoted by M. Attalides, Cyprus: Nationalism, p. 178, point 85.
137. Interview in *The Middle East*, September-October 1974, no. 3.
138. Oberling, op. cit., p. 184.
139. Ryan, op. cit., p. 198.
140. Callaghan, op. cit., p. 351.
141. Ibid., p. 354.
142. Polyvious, *Cyprus: Conflict*, p. 157.
143. Kaloudis, op. cit., p. 103.
144. Ibid., p. 107.
145. *UN Doc.* S/12723, 31 May 1978, para. 76.
146. *UN Doc.* S/11900, 8 December 1975, para. 16.
147. Van Coufoudakis, 'United Nations Peacekeeping and Peacemaking and the Cyprus Question', *Western Political Quarterly*, 29 (3), 1976, p. 470.
148. 'The Cyprus Dispute and the Search for a Settlement', *Australian Foreign Affairs Record*, October 1977, p. 501.
149. *A Study Mission Report*, 93rd Congress, 2nd session, 14 October 1974, p. 40.

6

INTERNATIONAL PEACEMAKING IN CYPRUS, 1980-1986

An outline survey

In 1980-6 a number of initiatives were launched by the United Nations to bring about a peaceful settlement to the Cyprus problem. This was largely owing to the appointment in 1982 of Javier Pérez de Cuéllar as UN Secretary-General. Having served as the special representative of his predecessor in Cyprus in the 1970s, the new Secretary-General was fully aware of the complexities and intricacies of the protracted dispute and was eager to find a satisfactory solution. Here each initiative will be considered together with the response of the two Cypriot communities. There were no independent initiatives by any other organisation or country in this period, although deliberations took place over various UN initiatives concerning Cyprus between the two Cypriot communities and their mother-countries. These are also dealt with in this chapter, since they played a part in the peacemaking process. Meanwhile, the West and the Soviet Union generally maintained the same attitude towards the problem as they had in the previous years, although the United States showed renewed interest in a settlement; their positions will also be discussed.

UNITED NATIONS PEACEMAKING IN CYPRUS, 1980-1986

The 'Interim Agreement' proposal

The first UN initiative during this period came from Secretary-General Waldheim in the fall and winter of 1980-1. This proposed an Interim Agreement between the disputants calling for, *inter alia*, the reopening of Nicosia's international airport to civilian traffic, the placing of Varosha under UN administration, and the lifting of some 70 per cent of the economic restrictions imposed by the Republic of Cyprus on the Turkish Cypriots.[1] The proposal was the result of a series of intercommunal talks, starting on 9 August 1980, under the auspices of the UN Secretary-

General's special representative in Cyprus, Ambassador Hugo Juan Gobbi. The two communities were represented at the talks by George Ioannides for the Greek Cypriots, and Umit Suleyman Onan for the Turkish Cypriots. In an 'opening statement' produced by the Secretary-General and read by Ambassador Gobbi at the start of the talks, the common ground between the two communities was stated to be the following:

(1) Both parties have reaffirmed the validity of the high-level agreements of 12 February 1977 and 19 May 1979;[2]
(2) Both parties have reaffirmed their support for a federal solution of the constitutional aspect and a bizonal solution of the territorial aspect of the Cyprus problem;
(3) Both parties have indicated that the matter of security can be raised and discussed in the intercommunal talks. It is understood that this matter will be discussed, having regard to certain practical difficulties which may arise for the Turkish Cypriot community, as well as to the security of Cyprus as a whole;
(4) Both parties have appealed to the Secretary-General for the continuation of the intercommunal talks.[3]

The 'Opening Statement' also referred to four subjects to be discussed at the intercommunal talks on the basis of 19 May 1979 agreement:

(1) reaching agreement on the resettlement of Varosha under United Nations auspices, in accordance with the provisions of point 5 of the 19 May agreement;
(2) initial practical measures by both sides to promote goodwill, mutual confidence and the return to normal conditions, in accordance with the provisions of point 6, which states that special importance will be given to this matter;
(3) constitutional aspects; and
(4) territorial aspects.[4]

It was decided at the end of the formal opening session to adjourn the talks till 16 September 1980. It was also agreed that the contents of the talks be kept private and confidential. While they were in progress the two interlocutors met, almost weekly, under the auspices of the Secretary-General's special representative, at the UN conference area at the Ledra Palace Hotel in Nicosia. They tackled the four items mentioned above in succession till 2 April 1981, when they announced that they would reduce the number of meetings during May and June while elections were held in both parts of Cyprus.[5] In his twice-yearly comprehensive report to the Security Council on all aspects of the UN operation in Cyprus, the Secretary-General stated on 27 May 1981:

> At the present stage, I have been given reason to believe that both parties may be prepared to make an intensive effort in the direction of a comprehensive settlement, involving the interconnected consideration of the territorial and constitutional aspects.[6]

The Greek-Cypriot attitude to the 'Interim Agreement' proposal. The attitude of the Greek Cypriots to this proposal, and the negotiations that followed on 9 August 1980, reflected the views of the government of Cyprus at the time. Spyros Kyprianou, then president of Cyprus, though officially supporting the Interim Agreement (which also initially enjoyed the support of his foreign minister, Nicos Rolandis), rejected the proposal.[7]

On entering into negotiations, the Greek Cypriots stated firmly that the procedure of the talks should on no account be interpreted as a modification of the two High-Level Agreements of 1977 and 1979. They also stressed that they were seeking a federal solution for the Cyprus problem, as envisaged in the 1977 and 1979 agreements. In their view, the federal state would comprise two federated states, one to be administered by the Greek Cypriots and the other by the Turkish Cypriots. The federal state, according to them, would be based on the accepted principles of federalism; there would be no border between the two regions and the central government would need to have sufficient power to ensure its unity. As a concession to the Turkish Cypriots, they accepted bi-regionality instead of multi-regionality which had been their original position. Subsequently the term 'bizonal' was used by the Greek-Cypriot side – the government of Cyprus – as a synonym for 'biregional' and in contrast to 'multiregional'. This term proved to be a controversial issue as the Greek Cypriots asserted that the Turkish Cypriot side had attached a different interpretation to the term than was originally accepted, as in an interview given by the Turkish Cypriot leader Rauf Denktash:

> The meaning of 'bizonal' is that I am a state that has territory as one of the two federated states. I am sovereign on many things within this territory. My sovereignty is absolute; no one can take it away from me.[8]

It therefore seems that the difference between the two sides at this stage was that the Greek Cypriots wanted a federation and the Turkish Cypriots a confederation. This created a wide gap between the two sides because the implications of each solution was quite different. President Kyprianou said at the beginning of the talks:

> Our target is a solution to the Cyprus problem, a solution of biregional federation, in all its aspects ... the word bi-zonal refers in this case to the territorial aspect only. [...] It would be inconceivable to have a partition federation. [...] Therefore, it is not at all correct to say that we have accepted bizonality.[9]

The different interpretations of the word 'bizonal' was the reason the Greek Cypriots could not agree to a settlement at this stage.

The Turkish-Cypriot attitude to the 'Interim Agreement' proposal. Throughout the 1980s the Turkish Cypriots were under the leadership of Rauf Denktash, a fact very much reflected in the intercommunal talks and in the attitude of Turkish Cypriots to the Interim Agreement proposal. The fundamental issue for the Turkish Cypriot leadership was the nature of the federal government in any given proposal. It argued that 'federation must be built from the basis of the existing two *de facto* administrations and that Cyprus should be a "decentralised" or "weak", federation with provisions for slow and long-term progress to a customs union and centralised fiscal and economic policy-making.'[10] Obviously, this differed widely from the Greek Cypriots' idea of a centralised federation, which Turkish Cypriots asserted was not a genuine 'federation', because a strong central government would have powers to override the units.[11] This difference sometimes showed itself in a bitter fashion: at one stage Denktash called his opposite number Kyprianou 'a shortsighted *Enosis* puppet', lacking all qualities of seriousness, responsibility and understanding.[12]

The 'Gobbi Initiative'

Despite the optimism of Secretary-General Waldheim, his proposed Interim Agreement did not produce the breakthrough he hoped for. However, it paved the way for another initiative devised by his special representative in Cyprus, Hugo Gobbi.[13] The Gobbi Initiative of 22 October 1981 was officially sent to the parties in dispute a month later, on 18 November. Although this initiative also failed to bring about a peaceful settlement, it was significant in that it became a basis for later negotiations between the two communities. Indeed, all negotiations from October 1981 to January 1983 were based directly on it. No official release concerning this initiative was ever made, and all deliberations took place behind closed doors. These negotiations gave rise to the terms 'points of equidistance' and 'points of coincidence', the latter being those points where there was an approximate coincidence of views, and the former where a median position existed on various subjects between quite divergent standpoints (see Appendix A).[14]

On his appointment as UN Secretary-General, Pérez de Cuellar found it useful to have frequent top-level meetings with the leaders of the two Cypriot communities – in April 1982 in Geneva, he met both Kyprianou and Denktash believing that the intercommunal talks were the best available method of continuing the negotiating process.[16] He also maintained direct contact with the governments of Greece and Turkey, meeting their foreign ministers in New York between June and October 1982.[17]

On 1 December 1982, the intercommunal talks were adjourned till 4 January 1983 for the annual recess; however, they subsequently suffered from the Turkish-Cypriots' disappointment with the Cyprus government's recourse to the General Assembly in May 1983, which led to Resolution 37/253 demanding 'the immediate withdrawal of all occupation forces from the Republic of Cyprus'.[18] Nevertheless, the negotiations based on the Gobbi initiative allowed a number of proposals and counter-proposals to be exchanged between the two communities. Owing to the confidentiality of most of those proposals and their frequency, they cannot be outlined in full, but they dealt with the resettlement of Varosha, the promotion of goodwill gestures, the constitutional aspect and the territorial aspect.

The Greek Cypriot attitude to the 'Gobbi Initiative'. Because of the confidentiality of the negotiations, it is difficult to say precisely what the Greek Cypriot response was to every item in the Gobbi initiative, but the main obstacle was clearly the nature of the federation, particularly the interpretation of the term 'bizonality'. As the Press and Information Office of the Government of Cyprus (the Greek Cypriot side) put it,

> The Turkish Cypriot side insisted on partition through the establishment of two separate administrations under a loose federal system. Furthermore the Turkish Cypriot side indicated that it was not prepared to relinquish any significant part of the territory under occupation. The Turkish Cypriot leadership gave clear evidence of its intention to consolidate the faits accomplis rather than seek a solution, when in July 1982 it decided to grant Turkish Cypriots and settlers from Anatolia title deeds to Greek Cypriot property.[19]

By resorting to the General Assembly[20] the Cyprus government aimed in part to apply pressure on the Turkish Cypriot leadership; the resulting resolution was a reminder of the international standing of the Greek Cypriots, the strongest leverage they have had in the negotiations.

The Turkish Cypriot attitude to the 'Gobbi Initiative'. The Turkish Cypriot response to the Gobbi initiative was in some ways different from that of the Greek Cypriots. The difference stemmed from the fact that Ambassador Gobbi approached the territorial aspect by tracing a line on the map of Cyprus with his finger,[21] which allowed each side to interpret the 'Gobbi line' as it desired. The Turkish Cypriots were firm about their interpretation and were reported to have accepted that aspect,[22] but there is no public record of the official response of either side.

'The Initiative'

In August 1983 a proposal, believed to have been drafted by the Secretary-General himself[23] and usually referred to as 'the Initiative' (also as 'indicators', 'soundings', 'parameters' or 'aide-memoires') was officially sent to the disputants.[24] According to its alleged text printed by a Cyprus newspaper,[25] the Initiative made some fundamental proposals. First it suggested the idea of a rotating presidency whereby Turkish Cypriots could, like the Greek Cypriots, aspire to the headship of a reunified Cypriot state. Secondly, unlike in the 1960 Constitution, the legislature was to be bicameral rather than unicameral. The lower chamber was to have representatives of the two communities in proportion to their population, while upper chamber would host an equal number of representatives from each community. Each community would vote for its own members in the parliament. Thirdly, concerning the executive branch of a reunified Cyprus, the Initiative proposed a ratio of 60 per cent Greek Cypriots to 40 per cent Turkish Cypriots as against the 70:30 ratio in the 1960 Constitution. The amount of territory to be given back by the Turks would be 8-13 per cent, reducing the existing 37 per cent to either 29 or 24 per cent. What the Initiative amounted to, according to the newspaper, was that 'the Turks would hand back some territory now under their control, while the Greek side surrendered governmental powers now in their hands.'[26]

The Greek-Cypriot attitude to 'the Initiative'. After initial signs to the contrary, the Initiative was eventually rejected by the Greek Cypriots, but not before it had caused a rift in the Cyprus government that led to the resignation of its foreign minister, Nicos Rolandis. Spyros Kyprianou remained in office following the presidential election on 13 February 1983.

The ruling party, DIKO, complained that the proposal failed to recognise the three basic freedoms which are the inalienable rights of every human being – right to free movement, right of settlement and right to property – throughout the island for all Cypriots. The party argued that such rights are contained in the Universal Declaration of Human Rights and could not be dispensed with in Cyprus. The 180,000 Greek Cypriot refugees, they said, should have the right to go back to their homes and live in their ancestral properties if they wished to do so. President Kyprianou himself was said to be 'lukewarm' towards the Initiative,[27] while the foreign minister Rolandis was 'enthusiastic'[28]. After much contention within the Greek Cypriot ranks, in which Greece allegedly played a part,[29] the Cyprus government came out against the Initiative and Rolandis offered his resignation on 20 September 1983. This led to a public war of words between him and the Cyprus government, in which he allegedly complained that 'Mr Kyprianou [did] not want meaningful negotiations on the problem of Cyprus'.[30]

The Turkish Cypriot Unilateral Declaration of Independence (UDI)

The Turkish Cypriot leader Rauf Denktash flew to New York on 30 September 1983, and after talks with the Secretary-General on the Initiative expressed his wish to have a high-level meeting with President Kyprianou, to which the Greek Cypriot leader responded positively. The aim of the meeting, according to Turkish Cypriots, was to 'clarify the position of the two sides'.[31] Barely a week later, however, the Initiative was stopped in its tracks by the Unilateral Declaration of Independence (UDI) by the Turkish Cypriot leadership, on 15 November.[32] The TFSC (Turkish Federated State of Cyprus) of 13 February 1975 was thus changed to the TRNC (Turkish Republic of Northern Cyprus). The UDI dealt a devastating blow to UN peacemaking efforts, and provoked strong reactions from the Greek Cypriots and the United Nations. In his letter to the Secretary-General dated 15 November 1983, Denktash professed a conviction that the proclamation of the Turkish Republic of Northern Cyprus will not hinder, but facilitate the re-establishment of the partnership between the two peoples within a federal framework',[33] adding that he 'sincerely desire[d] the continuation of Your Excellency's mission of good offices'.[34]

The United Nations reaction to the UDI. However, in resolution 541 of 18 November 1983, the UN Security Council forcefully rejected the UDI[35] stating that it 'deplores the Declaration of the Turkish Cypriot authorities of the purported secession of the part of the Republic of Cyprus'; that it 'considers the Declaration referred to above as legally invalid and calls for its withdrawal'; and also 'calls upon all states not to recognise any Cypriot state other than the Republic of Cyprus'.

The Security Council again asked the Secretary-General to pursue his mission of good offices 'in order to achieve the earliest possible progress towards a just and lasting settlement in Cyprus'.

The Greek Cypriot reaction to the UDI. Not surprisingly, the Greek Cypriot response to the UDI was vehement. In an immediate statement on the day it took place, President Kyprianou claimed that the action

> 'not only complicated further the Cyprus problem but made it clear that the intention of the Turkish side was always to create *faits accomplis* and to create conditions for the secession of the occupied area from the Republic of Cyprus.'[36]

The Greek Cypriots asserted that the UDI not only violated the sovereignty, independence and territorial integrity of Cyprus but was also against the UN Charter, the Helsinki Final Act and international law.[37]

Vienna 'Working Points' proposed by the Secretary-General

After his Initiative had failed as the result of UDI by the Turkish Cypriot leadership, Secretary-General Pérez de Cuéllar had meetings with the leaders of the two communities in the second half of November 1983, and in the same period also met the foreign ministers of Greece and Turkey, Messrs Haralambopoulos and Turkmen. In all his contacts the Secretary-General stressed to the parties the provisions of Security Council Resolution 541 and urged them to cooperate fully with him in attempting to bring about a peaceful settlement.[38]

On 11 January 1984 President Kyprianou presented a document to the Secretary-General, containing six sections, as a proposal for a settlement. This plan, initially intended by the Greek Cypriot leadership to be top secret, eventually found its way to the press.[39] It proposed the demilitarisation of Cyprus, an international force under UN auspices (with troops from countries not involved in the dispute) to maintain peace and security, international guarantees with no interested country as a party to the guarantee, and a genuine federation. It also allowed for territorial concessions to be made to the Turkish Cypriots allocating 25 per cent of the land to be under their control, provided that Famagusta in the east and Morphou in the north were returned to the Greek Cypriots. Finally, the document asked for a workable constitution, which the plan elaborated as follows:

(1) A Greek-Cypriot president and a Turkish-Cypriot vice-president; a council of ministers with 70:30 ratio of Greek Cypriots to Turkish Cypriots.
(2) Unicameral legislature preferred to a bicameral one; if the latter were adopted, a lower chamber with proportional representation of the two communities and an upper chamber with representation depending on the functions of the chamber.
(3) A federal supreme court, with equal representation of the two communities.
(4) The federal government to have powers over foreign affairs, international communications, passports, customs and tariffs etc.
(5) The three freedoms of movement, settlement and right to property to be secured throughout the country.

On receiving Kyprianou's framework proposals, the Secretary-General discussed a summary of them with Denktash. When Denktash complained that he should have been given a full text of Kyprianou's proposals, Pérez de Cuéllar said:

> 'I know that you would reject it totally, and it is not my purpose to give parties what they will reject; I try to find something that they could accept. That is why I did not give it to you.'[40]

On 16 March 1984 the Secretary General met Denktash in New York, and during their discussions asked him to stop the consolidation of TRNC and refrain from seeking recognition for it.[41] He also had talks with the Cyprus foreign minister, George Iacovou, on 19 and 20 March.

These meetings were intended to revitalise the intercommunal talks, which had been frozen since the Turkish Cypriot UDI, and were given substance by the following five-point plan (quoted verbatim):

(1) No further step to internationalise the Cyprus problem will be undertaken, and initiatives now underway will not be pursued.
(2) There will be no follow-up to 15 November 1983 declaration by the Turkish Cypriots, and initiatives currently underway would not be pursued.
(3) Both sides will make reciprocal commitments to the Secretary-General not to increase qualitatively or quantitatively the military forces in the island. They would also agree to a system of verification inspections by UNFICYP.
(4) The Turkish Cypriot authorities will transfer the Varosha area...to the Secretary-General, who will place it under interim United Nations administration, as part of the buffer zone controlled by UNFICYP. The transfer will be effected in phases over a period of six to nine months, to be agreed upon between His Excellency, Mr Denktash, and the Secretary-General and announced at the time of a high-level meeting.[...] It is understood that the area will not revert to the jurisdiction of the Greek Cypriots until a final agreement on a settlement of the Cyprus problem has been reached. No armed personnel other than UNFICYP will have access to this area.
(5) The parties will agree to accept a call by the Secretary-General for the holding of a high-level meeting and to the reopening of the intercommunal dialogue.[42]

These proposals failed to win the support of the Turkish Cypriot leadership. The Secretary-General's next move was to present on 7 August 1984 in Vienna, a set of ideas known as the Vienna Working Points to the representatives of the two communities, Messrs Mavromatis and Ertekun. According to press leaks[43] the Vienna Working Points consisted of the following items:

(1) Famagusta to be put under UN control and the eventual return of Greek Cypriots to their homes in that city.
(2) Reopening of Nicosia's international airport for use by both communities. This would be done under UN auspices but under Cypriot (both communities) administration.
(3) An immediate end to any further internationalisation of the Cyprus problem by the Greek Cypriots and a simultaneous stop to Turkish Cypriots seeking recognition for TRNC.
(4) Firm commitment by the leadership of both communities to the acceptance of the High-Level Agreements of 1977 and 1979.
(5) Agreement by both sides that a transitional government would implement any agreement reached and also work out the details of the federal constitution.

The Secretary-General was also said to have asked the two sides to consider four questions:

(1) Do the two communities agree to discuss the Working Points?
(2) If the Working Points are agreeable to both sides, would they therefore accept talks under his auspices towards an agreement?

(3) Should the talks prove successful, would the two leaders be prepared for a summit meeting?
(4) In case of agreement with the above items, would the first week of September be convenient to the two sides for the commencement of the talks?[44]

After much domestic political manoeuvring, mainly by the Greek Cypriots, both sides responded positively. The way was now open for further progress through what were to be known as the Proximity Talks.

The Greek-Cypriot attitude to the Vienna 'Working Points'. After the UDI by the Turkish Cypriot leadership, the Greek Cypriot's disappointment showed itself in various statements by the government of Cyprus. All the same, their overall attitude to the UN and its peacemaking efforts remained positive. Its most vociferous supporter was the communist party AKEL, operating south of the Green Line that marks the north-South divide in Nicosia between the two communities. At that time, the ruling party, DIKO, relied on AKEL's support in the parliament under a pact called the 'minimum programme'.

On 16 August 1984, after the questions had been put to the disputing parties by the Secretary-General for consideration, the foreign minister of Cyprus declared publicly that granting any more concessions to the Turkish Cyprist side would be tantamount to a 'slow death under the illusion of salvation'.[45] However, President Kyprianou consulted the Greek government as well as leaders of political parties at home on the Secretary-General's latest initiative. According to a Greek Cypriot daily, the president asked the Secretary-General to postpone a planned trip to Cyprus in September;[16] it can only be guessed that Kyprianou was under conflicting pressure from various political groups that prolonged his indecision over the Working Points. His eventual positive response, however, merely meant that the Greek Cypriot side was prepared to discuss the Working Points but not necessarily accept them as they stood.

The Turkish Cypriots' attitude to the Vienna 'Working Points'. The Turkish Cypriot side gave a positive response to the Working Points and the questions put down by the Secretary-General. Their response, accepting the initiative, came first on 7 August 1984 from Ertekun[47] and was later reaffirmed on 31 August.

'Proximity Talks'

On 10 September 1984 Proximity Talks began in New York. They were conducted in three rounds and led to the High-Level Summit of January 1985 in New York between Kyprianou and Denktash. They were held under the auspices of the UN and directly involved the

Secretary-General, who acted as the go-between and met the two delegations separately throughout; they led to the Secretary-General devising a 'draft agreement' which was eventually refused. It should be noted that the Vienna Working Points, which had led to the Proximity Talks, did not bind the parties as to what the Talks should contain; rather they covered the whole range of issues related to the Cyprus problem.

The first round of the Proximity Talks began on 10 September 1984 and lasted for ten days till 20 September. The Secretary-General suggested three headings for discussion: confidence-building measures, the structure of the federal government, and territorial adjustments. He also proposed a re-commitment of the two sides to the High-Level Agreements of 1977 and 1979 and the points agreed during intercommunal talks,[48] and recommended that the negotiations be kept confidential. This did not prevent leaks: two days after the start, a Greek Cypriot newspaper reported that the Secretary-General had proposed the reopening of Nicosia's international airport and the rehousing of the Greek Cypriots in the city of Famagusta under the heading of confidence-building measures and under UN auspices.[49] The substance of the Cyprus problem and the structure of the federal government were also discussed. Every aspect of the problem, including the three freedoms of movement, settlement and ownership received the attention of the two parties. This first round was rather complicated, with discussion on every small detail concerning the federal government and constitutional matters. Perhaps a more general outlook at this stage would have served the purpose better; at any rate, not much progress was made[50] and the negotiations halted on 20 September. The Secretary-General, however, described the first round as 'thorough and businesslike'.[51]

The second round began on 15 October and ended eleven days later. The agenda was set by the Secretary-General and again, though meant to remain confidential, somehow leaked to the press.[52] According to the leak, the agenda comprised two levels, one stating the points already agreed and the other describing the points to be agreed. The points already agreed by the parties included acceptance of the 1977 and 1979 High-Level Agreements, and the establishment at the earliest date of the federal republic of Cyprus, to be bicommunal in its the constitution and bizonal in its territory. It also included acceptance of those constitutional points already agreed in the 1981-3 intercommunal meetings: international representation of the Republic to be the function of the federal government, sovereignty to be exercised by the federal government on behalf both federated states and their respective territories, and the agreement on single citizenship afforded by the federal government. Points to be agreed were the powers and functions of the central government such as federal finance, foreign affairs, international transport, post and communications, defence and security, federal health and the federal judiciary. The proposed agenda called for a bicameral legislature with the upper chamber on a 50:50 ratio, and the lower chamber on a 70:30 ratio in favour of the Greek Cypriots. It also called for equal political status between the president and the vice-president. To resolve differences relating to the functions and powers of the federal government and the federated state, the agenda provided that a tripartite body with one non-Cypriot member be set up. As for the three freedoms (movement, settlement, right to property), the agenda asked for the establishment of working groups to deal appropriately with them and matters arising from them. The main difference between the parties seems to have been on the powers and functions of the central government. Nevertheless, the Secretary-General announced at the end of the second round that substantive progress had been achieved.[53]

The third and final round began on 26 November. The Secretary-General had asked the parties to come with their final positions and now presented them with a 'draft agreement' to be agreed upon at a subsequent high-level meeting. This bore similarities with the 1960 constitution with the main difference being, of course, that it was based on federalism.[54] The main points were a bicameral legislature consisting of an upper chamber (50:50 basis) and a lower chamber (70:30 basis), a Greek Cypriot president and a Turkish Cypriot vice-president, a cabinet made up of seven Greek Cypriot and three Turkish Cypriot ministers, a constitutional court, and a territory designating 29 per cent of the island for the Turkish Cypriots.

On 29 November, a ten-day recess was declared. Between 10 and 12 December there were further talks in New York, and it was announced subsequently that a high-level meeting between Kyprianou and Denktash would take place on 17 January in New York. The Secretary-General, in his twice-yearly Report to the Security Council, expressed optimism regarding the prospect of an overall agreement,[55] and the Security Council praised his efforts.[56] When asked by the press about duration of the proposed summit, the Secretary-General replied that 'one hour would be enough' for him, but if both sides so wished he would be at their disposal for two or three days.[57] At the opening of the summit he told the participants:

> 'If you are determined to reach an agreement, a unique chance now exists. If this moment is lost, I am sure you will agree, it may not readily recur.'[58]

However, it failed to get the agreement of both sides on the 'draft agreement', each side claiming that there had been misunderstandings over its acceptance. On 20 January the summit officially ended without having achieved any progress. The Proximity Talks had ended in failure.

The Greek Cypriot attitude towards the 'Proximity Talks'. The Greek Cypriot leadership seemed from the beginning to be less optimistic than the Secretary-General about the outcome of the Talks, and at the end it was Kyprianou who refused to accept the draft agreement as it stood. For the Greek Cypriots the main objection seems to have been around the area of the powers and functions of the central government. At the end of the second round of talks, differences between the two sides remained on almost all aspects of the dispute. The Greek Cypriots disagreed with a rotating presidency as proposed by the Turkish Cypriot side. The question of the legislature was also contentious, and although a bicameral legislature had been accepted in principle by both sides, the powers and functions of the upper chamber were still very much undecided. On the question of the territory of the federated states, the Greek Cypriots insisted on 25 per cent of the land for the proposed Turkish Cypriot federated state, while the Turkish Cypriot leaders were adamant on a 30 per cent share.

Meanwhile, pessimism prevailed in the Greek Cypriot camp. Before the start of the third round of talks, Kyprianou was reported to have said that he could not be hopeful on the outcome, but that a pleasant surprise would be most welcome.[59] During the third round, he presented the Secretary-General with a number of suggestions on the preliminary draft that the Secretary-General had asked both parties to study. According to the Greek Cypriot daily newspaper *Avgi*, Kyprianou's suggestions included the following:[60]

(1) The cabinet to be of 70:30 ratio for Greek and Turkish Cypriots.
(2) The bicameral legislature: lower House 80:20 ratio for Greek and Turkish Cypriots and the upper House on the basis of 50:50.
(3) Passports to be issued by the central government.
(4) Territory given to the Turkish Cypriots to equal 25 per cent of Cyprus's territory.
(5) Turkish troops to be withdrawn after signing the agreement.
(6) The foreign ministry not to be permanently allocated to a Turkish Cypriot politician.
(7) Airports and ports to be under the control of the central government.
(8) 'Political equality' not to imply numerical equality of the two communities.

Kyprianou therefore went to New York with 'cautious optimism' saying 'This is perhaps the first time since 1974 that some optimism is justified. But there is still a lot of distance to be covered in order to reach an agreed framework of a solution to the Cyprus problem covering all its aspects.'[61]

The summit itself started with what some have called 'the theatrical handshake of the century',[62] but it failed to live up to its opening. The 'draft agreement' prepared by the Secretary-General for signature at the summit was referred to by a Greek Cypriot spokesman as a 'ghost paper'.[63] Kyprianou refused to sign it as it stood and the summit ended in failure.

According to the Greek Cypriot version of events, the summit was not intended to be a mere formality but rather a forum for further negotiations; they claimed that this had been made clear by the Secretary-General in advance[64] and blamed the Turkish Cypriot side for refusing to negotiate the points contained in the 'draft agreement'. Meanwhile, Kyprianou's refusal to sign the agreement brought him much criticism at home; he had been under pressure from the right-wing DISY and the communist AKEL to be more flexible. The former foreign minister Rolandis launched an attack with an open letter to the President:

> I am happy neither with the New York melodrama with its multitude of substantial statements, nor with the resulting confusion and misunderstanding... Have you not, by your actions at the proximity talks and after, opened the door for Denktash to create new *fait accomplis*? [...] You have no right to play on the future of Cyprus the unacceptable tricks you have played on the political parties.[65]

Some of the international press, as well as some of the Greek Cypriot press, also blamed the failure on President Kyprianou: according to *The Times* of London, 'UN officials said President Kyprianou even questioned the basic tenets and principles of an accommodation.' However, some believe that Kyprianou had every intention of coming to an agreement after an acceptable framework had been negotiated between the parties, and this would seem to be confirmed by his acceptance of the draft agreement at the eleventh hour, with the condition that another summit be held to negotiate four issues: withdrawal of Turkish troops from Cyprus, the three freedoms of movement, settlement and right to property, guarantor powers, and lastly the areas to be returned to the Greek Cypriots by the Turkish Cypriots.[66] The last point was apparently of the utmost importance to the Greek Cypriot side, since 'Kyprianou evidently staked the outcome of the talks on the exact location of the land to be returned'.[67]

It is difficult if not possible to determine for certain whether or not the failure of the Proximity Talks should be imputed to Kyprianou. He had expressed his reservations from the beginning and came to the summit with the aim of negotiating further. There was no immediate election in prospect for him at the time, which strengthened his position. What is certain is that his handling of the summit contributed to its failure and put good propaganda material into the hands of the Turkish Cypriots. As we shall see, Denktash was perhaps not enthusiastic for an agreement either, but if that is true, then Kyprianou played into his hands.[68]

The Turkish-Cypriot attitude to 'Proximity Talks'. On the surface, the Turkish Cypriot position in the Proximity Talks was clear. They accepted the Secretary-General's draft agreement 'as if' the Greek Cypriots would do so too.[69] If they did accept it, then negotiations could be expanded.[69] It should be noted that they accepted the whole document without exceptions. Denktash said that he had been promised by the Secretary-General that 'not even a comma of this paper can be altered without your consent and I shall be there to see that this is so. [...] The document is to be accepted as a whole or rejected.'[70] The sticking point was the question of the powers and functions of the central government, which the Turkish Cypriots insisted should evolve from the two existing regional administrations rather than the central authority devolving powers to the two regions.[71] In their view the question of territory and the exact areas allocated for each federated state, though important, was to be decided after agreement on other issues and on the basis of economic viability, land ownership and security.[72] .

It is difficult to know whether Denktash was genuine in accepting the draft agreement. The 'working points' which had initiated the Proximity Talks seemed to some observers to favour the Turkish Cypriots' position on central government.[73] Thus, basically, he had a good deal. But he was under pressure from Turkey to come to an agreement and to reject it could have proved costly to him. His wariness in the negotiations suggests that he accepted it only in anticipation that Kyprianou would reject it. One observer noted:

> In the Greek Cypriot view...shared by some well-placed diplomats, Mr Denktash is more inclined to consolidate his secession than to give anything more than lip-service to the effort to find a federal solution.[74]

If this was the case, Denktash played his hand well, refusing to accept Kyprianou's request for another summit on the grounds of the forthcoming Turkish-Cypriot elections. He had got out of a tight corner very successfully.

The 'Draft Framework Agreement'

Towards the end of 1985 and the beginning of 1986, the Secretary-General had meetings with both parties in London and Geneva to discuss points of convergence and tackle the points of divergence between the two sides.[75] On 29 March , he presented a new Draft Framework Agreement,[76] which was made public and was accompanied by a letter to the leaders of the two communities. The Secretary-General also sent copies to the permanent members of the Security Council as well as to Greece and Turkey. However, this initiative also failed to find an agreement acceptable to both sides. The 1986 Draft Framework Agreement was similar in many ways to the failed January 1985 summit proposals. However, it differed in tone on the uneasy formula equating the Greek Cypriots' concession over the powers of the central government with the Turkish-Cypriots' concession over the amount of territory they would part with. The issues of security and defence were left for later negotiations of new defence treaties. The legislature was to be the same as that proposed in January 1985, but important matters would require separate majorities for each community represented in the parliament. A working group was to be set up to discuss the three freedoms, and a timetable was to be agreed for the withdrawal of foreign troops. It was understood that the amount of territory to be given to the Turkish Cypriots was to be at least 29 per cent.

The Draft Framework Agreement was rejected by the Greek Cypriot side. The Secretary-General in his Report of 11 June to the Security Council regretted that, 'since one side is not yet in a position to accept the draft framework agreement of 29 March 1986, the way is not yet open to proceed with the negotiations I have proposed for an overall solution'.[77] In response to suggestions by the Cyprus government about convening an international conference on the Cyprus problem, an idea for which he had no mandate, the Secretary-General said he had told Kyprianou that the Security Council was divided on the matter.[78] Twenty-two years after the United Nations was first entrusted with the mission of bringing about a peaceful settlement for the island. The Cyprus problem had yet again proved impervious to his mission of good offices.

The Greek-Cypriot attitude to the 'Draft Framework Agreement'. The bitter criticism the Greek Cypriot leadership faced at home for its handling of the New York summit eased somewhat with their acceptance of the 'draft agreement' of April 1985. This was viewed as a concession[79] and following the Turkish Cypriot rejection of it, the Greek Cypriot leadership were reassured by the UN Secretariat that any new document would include only cosmetic changes and would not differ in substance. According to Greek Cypriots, however, the new Draft Framework Agreement ran contrary to such assurances. Their main objections were as follows:[80]

(1) It ignored the criterion of the number of refugees to return to their homes, thus blocking the way to a fair settlement of the territorial problem.
(2) It accorded full political equality to the Turkish Cypriot minority of 18 per cent with the Greek Cypriot majority of 80 per cent without the corresponding balance in the government structure.
(3) It provided for Turkish Cypriot vetoes on all matters both in the Executive and the Legislative, without adequate deadlock-resolving mechanisms.
(4) It provided for a separate international personality for the constituent members allowing them to act as sovereign states.

(5) It did not provide for an effective implementation of the three freedoms (movement, settlement, property ownership), which are essential attributes of citizenship in any state.
(6) It prescribed a predominantly confederal rather than a federal state.

On 20 April President Kyprianou wrote to the Secretary-General, citing three topics to be negotiated at a meeting between himself and Denktash: withdrawal of Turkish forces and settlers, effective international guarantees, and application of the three freedoms of movement, settlement and the right to property.[81] In a subsequent letter dated 10 June, he expressed his reservations as follows:

> When confronted with the proposals of the 'draft framework agreement' the concept of the integrated whole on its own is not sufficient protection for our position, as the Greek Cypriot side would find itself bound by unworkable constitutional and other arrangements prejudicial to it, without benefiting from any corresponding obligation on the part of the Turkish Cypriot leadership with regard to all those matters which are of vital concern to the Greek Cypriots.[82]

Other Greek Cypriot leaders were more direct, telling American reporters simply that the proposals should be scrapped.[83]

The Turkish Cypriot attitude to the 'Draft Framework Agreement'. The Turkish Cypriot leadership's response to the Draft Framework Agreement was positive,[84] possibly because it was now in a stronger position. During the preceding year, the Turkish Cypriot leadership had consolidated their declaration of a 'Turkish Republic of Northern Cyprus'. First, on 12 March 1985, their constitution was put to referendum and subsequently, on 23 June of the same year, parliamentary elections were held in the north of the island. These actions were essentially 'double edged'. On the one hand, they infuriated the Greek Cypriots and caused uproar among their press and politicians, boosting the position of radicals in the south. On the other hand, by opening up the prospect, however remote, of acquiring international recognition at some future date, they put pressure on the Greek Cypriots to grant further concessions. The Turkish Cypriots' earlier rejection of the 1985 draft agreement may have been the result of their unwillingness to negotiate before this process of consolidation had taken place. Whether the measures were taken merely to apply pressure on the Greek Cypriot side or to seek a separate political identity is still open to question. (Like President Kyprianou, Denktash was not immune to opposition at home, although opposition figures such as Ozker Ozgur, leader of the Turkish Republican Party were discriminated against quite strongly and suffered from persecution in the north of the island and hence tended to play a smaller role than their Greek Cypriot counterparts).

In response to Kyprianou's suggestion of a summit to discuss the withdrawal of Turkish troops, guarantees and the three freedoms, Denktash told the Secretary-General:

> The Turkish Cypriot side is definitely against any new procedures envisaging any form of secret or 'shuttle' diplomacy or any kind of summit meeting prior to the Greek Cypriot acceptance of the 'Draft Framework Agreement'. Such new procedures would clearly fall outside the scope of the integrated-whole character of the 'Draft framework agreement'.[85]

The issues that divided the two parties on the Draft Framework Agreement seem to have been precisely those that Kyprianou wanted to discuss. For Turkish Cypriots the only effective guarantee was provided by Turkey;[86] Turkish troops could not leave the island before the establishment of the transitional federal government without threatening their security. Nor, in their view, could the three freedoms be practised throughout the island without some sort of regulation. For the Greek Cypriots the reverse was the case. The events of 1974 demonstrated only too clearly that Turkey was the only country which could not be entrusted with any guarantee status whatever and Turkish troops should leave as soon as the agreement was signed, since their continued presence only increased tension by threatening the security of the Greek Cypriot community. In any case, the three freedoms were the inalienable rights of any citizen of any country in the world, embodied in the Universal Declaration of Human Rights; why make an exception in the case of Cyprus? These fundamentally opposite views could not be reconciled in the context of the Draft Framework Agreement, although the three freedoms were the issue that promised further progress, as both sides did show some sign of flexibility on the subject.

In November 1986, in a meeting at the Royal Institute of International Affairs (Chatham House) in London, Denktash reiterated his position concerning the Draft Framework Agreement, and said he would still be prepared to enter into negotiations with the Greek Cypriots on that basis.

OUTSIDE POWERS AND INTERNATIONAL PEACEMAKING IN CYPRUS, 1980-1986

The United Kingdom. During the 1980-6 period Britain's general attitude to the Cyprus problem, except in 1983, can best be described as one of inactivity. After the Conservative election victory in 1979, the issue was not even referred to in the parliamentary programme, despite protests from the back benchers, which seemed to indicate lack of interest.

However, the government continued to support the United Nations peacemaking efforts.

The government did respond decisively to the Turkish Cypriot UDI, requesting an urgent meeting of the Security Council and submitting a draft resolution (Resolution 541 of the Security Council of 1983) condemning the UDI and demanding its immediate withdrawal.[87] Britain's UN representative said that the British government recognised only the Cypriot state headed by President Kyprianou and that the Turkish action was 'incompatible with the state of affairs as brought about by the Treaties governing the establishment of the Republic of Cyprus'.[88] Following the adoption of this Resolution the British government proposed a tripartite conference in London between the guarantor powers Greece, Turkey and Britain. The proposal was rejected by the Greek government, which reportedly favoured parallel bipartite conferences between the Britain and each of the other two states.[89] The proposal for the tripartite conference was Britain's last active engagement in peacemaking in Cyprus in 1980-6, although it continued to maintain a contingent in the UN peacekeeping force there.

Generally, during this period, British policy consisted chiefly of support for the Secretary-General's efforts for a united Cyprus. The Prime Minister Margaret Thatcher said that she wished 'Cyprus to continue in a state of unity as it did nine years ago before it was rudely upset'.[90]

It can be argued that as long as its bases in Cyprus were not threatened, the British government lacked the incentive to launch a major peacemaking effort. On the other hand, the United States played a more active role during this period yet failed to achieve anything, and there could be no guarantee that a more energetic involvement on Britain's past would have borne fruit either. Nor did Britain's proposal for a conference receive universally positive response. Nonetheless, as a guarantor power, a more active engagement by Britain would have been a welcome development for the Greek and Turkish Cypriots alike.

Greece. The 1980-6 period continued to see the profound impact of Greek foreign policy over Cyprus, possibly greater even than in the aftermath of 1974 coup and the invasion. That is to say, the relations between Greece and Turkey affected the way Greece used its influence in Cyprus, to the extent that in 1986 the Greek Prime Minister Andreas Papandreou was accused by the United States of using Cyprus as part of his anti-Turkish policy, and of being the source of Greek Cypriot intransigence in the intercommunal negotiations.[91] Certainly, Cyprus was universally seen in Greece as an indication of Turkish intentions in the Aegean, with particular implications for the security of the Greek islands along the Turkish coast.[92]

The 1981 election of the Greek Socialist Party, PASOK had a direct impact on Cyprus. Its leader, Papandreou, was less flexible than his predecessor. In February 1982 he became the first Greek prime minister to visit Cyprus,[93] and later he supported Kyprianou in refusing to sign either the agreement at the summit of January 1985 or the Draft Framework Agreement of March 1986.[94] This negative attitude can be imputed to the Greek government's view of Turkey as the main enemy of Hellenism generally and, by extension, of Greece itself.[95] The close relations of the United States with Turkey on the one hand and the comparatively poor ones with Greece added to the Greek government's sense of insecurity in the face of an enemy that was militarily three times stronger than Greece. Because of this, some observers have seen Cyprus as stick with which Greece could beat Turkey at will.[96]

It can hardly be disputed that for most of the 1980-6 period Greece had difficult relations with the United States. It was the only EC country not to impose sanctions on Poland in the early 1980s when martial law was introduced there,[97] and the only NATO country not to approve the deployment of Pershing II and Cruise missiles in Europe.[98] Papandreou repeatedly stated his intention of closing all US bases in Greece by 1988 and refused to allow US marines to be resupplied at Greek ports.[99] The reason Papandreou's government did not withdraw Greece from NATO altogether was that this would only have enhanced Turkey's strategic significance even further.[100] Greece's poor relations with the United States made Greco-Turkish relations more confrontational in a situation where their common membership of the Atlantic Alliance afforded Greece the security of the big protector, the United States. Greek policy-makers were well aware that the United States could not afford to allow Turkey to engage in military conflict with Greece, hence their leverage with Cyprus.

Overall the Greek impact on peacemaking in Cyprus during this period was negative because of its bad relations with Turkey. As the stronger of the two countries, Turkey could not be allowed to extricate itself from Cyprus unscathed, depriving Greece of a useful stick with which to beat its old adversary; if nothing else, the issue could be exploited to block or reduce the US administration's aid to Turkey.

Turkey. Turkey's involvement continued on the same level as in the post-invasion period, dominated as before by the island's strategic importance and by the security of the Turkish Cypriots. In 1980 Turkey was suffering from chronic domestic violence: the monthly death toll had reached 200, double that of 1979, and there were said to be at least forty-seven terrorist factions roughly split between leftists on the one hand and separatists and religious or right-wing extremists on the other.[101] In September 1980 a military coup took place and martial law came into force; civilian rule was not restored till December 1983. This confusion had a negative effect on the peace process.

After the military takeover, General Evren, the new head of state, sent a message to the Turkish Cypriot leadership which described Cyprus as 'the daughter of the motherland' and 'an integral part of Turkey'.[102] On a visit to the TRNC in 1986, Turkey's prime minister Turgut Özal remarked: 'The moment I set foot here, I felt myself in one of the provinces, towns and villages of Turkey. There is no difference.'[103] Such statements reinforced suspicions in Greece and among Greek Cypriots of Turkish intentions, making the granting of concessions by the Greek Cypriots even more difficult. The tendency to treat Cyprus as part of Turkey also drew criticism from Turkish-Cypriot politicians; when Özal visited northern Cyprus, he came, the opposition leader Özker Ozgur said, 'not ... as a guest but as if he were the owner of the TRNC.'[104]

Turkey's control over the northern third of the island has indeed been extensive and multifaceted. In 1984, as in other years, Turkey provided two-thirds of its budget.[105] Militarily it has had full control since 1974, with some 40,000 troops stationed there, while in terms of communication it has been the only route to the outside world for northern Cyprus because of the international boycott of the TRNC. Even in Turkish Cypriot internal politics Turkey continued to play a dominant role in the 1980-6 period for instance interfering directly in leadership elections in Denktash's National Unity Party.[106] As Turkey was the only country to extend recognition to the UDI, there can be little doubt that during this period it could have influenced Denktash, despite claims that he enjoyed considerable autonomy.[107]

However, like Greece, Turkey did not view the Cyprus problem in isolation but as an important bargaining counter in its differences with Greece over the Aegean. Also, as Turkey's relations with the West improved further in this period, it could be exploited for the fulfilment of its ambition to join the European Community, for example by offering concessions in exchange for a more welcoming posture. During the 1980-6 period, however, there was no move on either of these fronts, and Turkey therefore lacked any motive to yield on Cyprus. The only factor that might have persuaded it to make a move on the Cyprus problem was its dependence on the West, and the impact of the problem on the assistance it received from that quarter. For instance, in March 1984 the US Senate Foreign Relations Committee voted to withhold $215m in military aid unless Turkey handed over control of Famagusta to the UN.[108] However, such measures were ineffective: 'if they have tied the aid to concessions on Cyprus', the Turkish prime minister reported, 'then they are dreaming.'[109]

Perhaps the failure of such measures can be attributed to the strategic importance of Turkey and Turkey's own awareness of its significance. Besides controlling naval traffic through the Bosphorus, it straddles the air routes connecting the Soviet Union to the Middle East and is ideally placed to support Western intervention in the Persian Gulf.[110] The latter became particularly important after the Iranian Revolution in 1979 and the consequent loss by the United States of an important ally;[111] any undue pressure over Cyprus carried the risk of distancing Turkey from the West, which the West could not afford. A visit by General Evren to Bulgaria, Romania and Yugoslavia in 1982, together with a visit to Moscow by the Turkish foreign minister earlier in the same year, had shown that Turkey was capable of forging closer ties with the East. So Turkish policy-makers could be confident that sticking to their guns over Cyprus would not greatly jeopardise assistance from the West, particularly as the Reagan administration had adopted a pro-Turkish policy.

Overall, the 1980-6 period was disappointing where the Turkish attitude to peacemaking in Cyprus was concerned. Although officially it paid lip-service to intercommunal negotiations[112] its actions tended to go in the opposite direction. Certainly, Turkey knew well in advance about the UDI and supported it,[113] in spite of the fact that it effectively ended the 1983 UN Initiative.[114] Cyprus was too important an issue for Turkey to yield on without gaining concessions in the Aegean or over EC membership. It could not add to the insecurity of a ring of Greek islands threatening its Western coast by withdrawing its troops from a large island a mere 40 miles away where, moreover, communist influence was strong.[115]

One Turkish diplomat said to a Greek counterpart in the late 1980s, 'We have won in Cyprus, it is just a matter of time for you to realise it.'[116]

The United States. In the 1980-6 period the US attitude to the Cyprus problem showed a marked difference compared to the past,[117] with Washington being more active in trying to bring a peaceful end to the conflict. The geo-strategic significance of the island had been enhanced with the advances of Soviet influence in the region[118] and the corresponding decline of US influence in the early 1980s.[119] The minimum requirement for the State Department was that the Cyprus problem should not be allowed to escalate into a Greco-Turkish war since both countries were members of NATO.

The change in emphasis arose out of three considerations associated with Cold War diplomacy:[120] helping the US build a stronger NATO, Cyprus being within the Western sphere of influence; alleviating the prospect of a Greco-Turkish conflict; and removing domestic opposition to further military aid to Turkey, which Congress held responsible for the impasse. An example of this was seen in 1984 when the shift in US policy over Cyprus manifested itself in the High-Level Summit of January 1985 between the two community leaders in New York. Earlier, on 22 November 1984, President Reagan had sent a letter to his Turkish counterpart, General Kenan Evren, asking him to apply pressure on Denktash for more flexibility.[121] Partly as the result of this the leaders of the two communities in Cyprus met in January 1985, for the first time in six years. The United States also showed interest in the UN peacemaking efforts, sending a State Department counsel, Edward J. Derwinski, to Cyprus to help out. The US government rounded off these diplomatic moves with the offer to Cyprus of a $250 million grant in the event of a breakthrough.[122] All this was applauded by the Greek Cypriots.[123]

As before, US policy during this period was dictated by Cold War considerations: containment of the aggressive Soviet military and political posture in the region required careful and firm planning. According to a report in 1984, the Warsaw Pact forces could 'operate anywhere in the Mediterranean, endangering the security of sea lines of communication which are of vital importance to the NATO nations in the Southern Flank.'[124] In planning and implementing an effective strategy to combat the Soviets in the area, Cyprus played an important part,[125] through its location and the relatively large size of its geographical area and its population on the one hand, and its ability to create tensions on the other.[126]

To be in a position to bring about a solution to the Cyprus problem, the US government had to have good relations with the two mother-countries, Greece and Turkey, whose influence in their respective communities in Cyprus was considerable. A factor was the presence in the United States of about 1.25 million Greek Americans and 54,000 Turkish Americans,[127] although the influence of the Greek lobby in Washington tended to be outweighed by Turkey's strategic significance as one of the two NATO countries (Norway being the other) to have a border with the Soviet Union, with 630,000 soldiers ready to fight under Alliance command. But while Turkey enjoyed support in the Pentagon, the presence of its troops in Cyprus in violation of international law caused the State Department to support Greece.[128]

During the 1980s US relations with Turkey warmed, with President Reagan's election and the coming to power of the military government in Turkey, both of which led to a strengthening of military and commercial ties. As Helen Laipson writes,

> The military government that ruled Turkey from September 1980 until elections in 1983 won favour in Reagan's camp, both because of its anti-Soviet stance and because it came to power in a life-and-death struggle against terrorism. The 1983 election of Turgut

> Özal to the Premiership further strengthened the bonds, based on shared strategic and economic philosophies.[129]

The amount of US aid to Turkey increased dramatically between 1982 and 1983,[130] and trade between the two countries also grew substantially.[131] All this meant that the United States had more influence in Turkey, which helped to bring about the 1985 New York summit between the two Cypriot leaders.

US relations with Greece took a turn for the worse following the election of the socialist government in 1981, reaching their nadir in June 1985 when the US government issued travel advice to its citizens warning that it no longer had faith in the Greek government's anti-terrorist efforts, and considered Athens airport unsafe for travellers.[132] Ironically, this warning acted as a spur to improved relations between the two countries, and the following month the warning was withdrawn. However, US relations with Greece during the first seven years of the 1980s never had the significance and warmth of those with Turkey.

In view of America's willingness to use its influence with Greece and Turkey and its encouragement and support for UN efforts, why was the Cyprus conflict not settled in this period? Without its support no solution could have been be envisaged.[133] The answer to this question is twofold. First, the extent of US influence in Greece and Turkey should not be overestimated, and secondly, the American perception of the Cyprus problem suffered from certain inadequacies.

The amicable relations between the United States and Turkey in 1980-6 were mutually beneficial: the United States strengthened the Atlantic Alliance, and Turkey built up its military and its poor economy with American aid. Any worsening of relations would have been detrimental to both countries; thus US leverage with Turkey over the Cyprus problem was limited, and 'heavy-handed pressure could backfire'.[134] As for Greece, the socialist government of Papandreou was not particularly amenable to pressures from the United States, and there too, US influence was limited. Another limiting factor was US policy-makers' perception of the Cyprus problem as basically an intercommunal dispute rather than, as Leigh Bruce put it the result of '30 years of shortsighted policy and manipulation by outside powers – Great Britain, Greece, Turkey, and the United States'.[135] Underestimating the international aspect, perhaps the most important aspect of the Cyprus problem,[136] hampered US efforts to bring about a peaceful settlement to the conflict. However, none of these factors – the limited influence of the United States with Turkey and Greece, and its perception of the Cyprus problem as primarily an intercommunal one – altered the fact that the United States was the only actor with sufficient leverage to influence all the parties to the problem. Meanwhile, its support for the UN peacemaking efforts, though half-hearted at times,[137] was more forthcoming in this period than in the preceding ones. The UN was still a forum where the Soviet Union could become a party in the making of a Cyprus solution, and as such it was viewed with some concern by the United States.

The Soviet Union. Soviet policy towards Cyprus in the 1980-6 period continued to be dominated by the Cold War. On the one hand, it continued to back the Cyprus government, as the representative of an independent and a non-aligned country; on the other, the strategic significance of Turkey meant that it would be open to persuasion by Turkey on Cyprus if Turkey ever decided to loosen its ties with the West. In turn, supporting the Cyprus government without completely closing its doors to Turkey was the thrust of the Soviet policy in this period.

Superpower rivalry and the policy of containment allowed smaller states to play a bigger role in international relations.[138] The significance of Cyprus in the sensitive eastern Mediterranean area was thus out of proportion to its size and population. All the guarantor countries of Cyprus – Britain, Greece and Turkey – were members of NATO, a fact that the Soviet Union never lost sight of. Because of this, and in line with its policy of supporting Cyprus's independence, sovereignty, non-alignment and territorial integrity, the Soviets supported all UN efforts to bring about a settlement, not wishing to see a partition that could lead eventually to what they termed 'Nato-isation' of the country. In their support of the UN Secretary-General's 1983 Initiative, they sent a high level foreign ministry delegation to Cyprus.[139] Later, on 21 January 1986, in an attempt to get more actively involved, the Soviet Union asked through its UN ambassador that an international conference on the Cyprus problem be convened. The Soviet proposals were entitled 'Principles of a Cyprus settlement and ways of achieving it', and were circulated among UN members.[140] The Greek Cypriots supported the proposal and have since asked for the convening of such a conference.

Soviet relations with Greece were friendly, but despite Papandreou's socialist government being in power for most of the 1980-6 period, and the cooling of relations between Greece and the United States, Greco-Soviet relations never reached a level that endangered Greek commitment to the Atlantic Alliance or could have enabled the Soviets to regard Greece as an ally. The Soviet stance on the Cyprus problem won praise from Greece, but it had not in any way managed to influence the Cyprus problem through Greece. As for Turkey, the Cyprus problem somewhat soured relations between the two countries in this period.[141] The coming to power of the military in Turkey pushed Turkey closer to the West, and as a result, Soviet policy makers had only limited leverage with Ankara even after it returned to civilian rule.

By supporting all relevant resolutions, the Soviet Union continued its support of the United Nations peacemaking efforts in Cyprus and tried to make as much capital as possible out of it against the West in general and the United States in particular. However, this support was not wholehearted, as was evident from the failure of the Eastern bloc to maintain its contributions towards the maintenance of the UN force in Cyprus.[142] The Soviet Union had little impact on the Cyprus problem as a whole, although its 1986 proposals for an international conference were supported by the Greek Cypriots and briefly complicated the Secretary-General's endeavours to find a solution to the Cyprus problem.[143]

During the 1980-6 period, the United Nations was more active in taking various initiatives to solve the Cyprus problem than in the preceding years. It can also be said that the United States was more supportive of these efforts of the UN than previously. Nonetheless a Cyprus settlement proved as elusive as ever. Intercommunal mistrust was more evident in the negotiations at this time than in previous years. The fear each side felt towards the intentions of the other was paramount in the 1980-6 negotiations. However, on balance the Turkish Cypriot side was less flexible than the Greek Cypriot side towards the peacemaking efforts.

With active US engagement in this period, the chances of a settlement were increased. However, Turkey's reluctance to apply sufficient pressure on Denktash contributed to the stalemate. Correspondingly, the hardline stance of Greece on the issue also had much to do with the failure. It seemed, somewhat strangely, that Greece, Turkey and the two communities in Cyprus were all unwilling to take any major steps towards a settlement. Perhaps they preferred to keep what they had rather than commit themselves to a settlement process, which in the end might prove unsatisfactory.

NOTES

1. See *UN Doc.* S/14275, 1st December 1980, para. 42.
2. For details of the two agreements see the previous chapter.
3. Annex to *UN Doc.* S/14100, 11 August 1980.
4. Ibid.
5. *UN Doc.* S/14490. 27 May 1981, para. 43.
6. Ibid., para. 57.
7. Glen, D. Camp, manuscript prepared for *Polity, Journal of the Northeast Political Science Association* (1988), p. 9.
8. Interview with the Turkish Cypriot Magazine *Olay* conducted on 16 July 1979.
9. Ertekun, *The Cyprus Dispute and the Birth of the Turkish Republic of Northern Cyprus* Nicosia: K. Rustem and Bro., 2nd Edition, 1984, appendix 59, pp. 370-1.

10. Zaim M. Necatigil, *The Cyprus Question and the Turkish Position in International Law*, Oxford University Press, 1989, p. 148.
11. Ibid., p. 149.
12. Ertekun, op. cit., appendix 60, p. 373.
13. For discussion of the Gobbi Initiative see *UN Doc.* S/15502, 1 December 1982, para. 47 and S/15149, 1 June 1982, para. 45.
14. See *UN Doc.* S/15812, 1 June 1983, p. 11, para. 49.
15. Ertekun, op. cit., p. 112.
16. *UN Doc.* S/15149, 1 June 1982, para. 55.
17. *UN Doc.* S/15502, 1 December 1982, para. 49.
18. See Appendix 2.
19. *The Cyprus Problem*, Nicosia: Press and Information Office, August 1987, p. 36.
20. See Appendix 2.
21. Source does not wish to be identified.
22. Camp, op. cit., p. 10.
23. Ibid., p. 10.
24. See Appendix 3.
25. *Cyprus Mail*, 18 August 1983.
26. Quoted by Camp, op. cit., p. 11.
27. Ibid., pp. 11-12.
28. Ibid.
29. Ibid.
30. Rauf R. Denktash, *The Cyprus Triangle*, Lefkosa: K. Rustem and Bro., 2nd edition, 1988, p. 278.
31. Ertekun, op. cit., p. 121.
32. For the text of the UDI see *UN Docs.* A/38/586 and S/16148, 16 November 1983, appendices B and C.
33. Ibid., appendix A.
34. Ibid.
35. See Appendix 4.
36. Quoted in *The Cyprus Problem* op. cit., pp. 39 and 40.
37. Ibid., p. 40.
38. *UN Doc.* S/16192, 1 December 1983, para. 57.
39. Athens paper *Nea*, 26 January 1984 (translation provided by Maria Mirbagheri).
40. Necatigil, op. cit., p. 214.
41. *Cyprus Mail*, 15 and 18 March 1984.
42. *UN Doc.* S/16519, 1 May 1984.
43. Greek-Cypriot daily *Agon*, 12 August 1984 (translation provided by Maria Mirbagheri).
44. Greek-Cypriot daily *Simerini*, 19 August 1984 (translation provided by Maria Mirbagheri).
45. *Cyprus Mail*, 17 August 1984.
46. Greek-Cypriot daily *Alithia*, 25 August 1984 (translation provided by Maria Mirbagheri).
47. Denktash, op. cit., p. 132.
48. See Greek-Cypriot daily *Alithia*, 12 September 1984 (translation provided by Maria Mirbagheri).
49. See Greek-Cypriot daily *Simerini*, 12 September 1984 (translation provided by Maria Mirbagheri).
50. See Greek-Cypriot dailies *Agon*, 16 September 1984, and *Phileleftheros*, 16 September 1984 (translation provided by Maria Mirbagheri).
51. Denktash, op. cit., p. 133.
52. See *Cyprus Mail*, 23 October 1984.
53. See *UN Press Release*, CYP/94/13, Nicosia.

54. *UN Doc.* S/16858, 12 December 1984, para. 50.
55. Ibid.
56. *UN Doc.* S/PV 2565, 14 December 1984.
57. Quoted by Denktash, op. cit., p. 137.
58. Ibid., appendix 26, p. 376.
59. *Cyprus Mail*, 27 November 1984.
60. Greek-Cypriot daily Avgi, 16 December 1984 (translation provided by Maria Mirbagheri).
61. Quoted in *The Cyprus Problem*, op cit., p. 45.
62. Quoted by Camp, op. cit., p. 21.
63. *The New York Times*, 21 January 1985.
64. See *The Cyprus Problem*, op. cit., p. 45.
65. Quoted by Denktash, op. cit., appendix 27, p. 377.
66. *Washington Post*, 21 January 1985.
67. Camp, op. cit., p. 22.
68. Ibid., p. 23.
69. Ibid., pp. 21 and 22.
70. Denktash, op. cit., p. 133.
71. Robert McDonald, 'Cyprus: the UN tries again', *The World Today*, vol. 40, no. 10, October 1984, p. 420.
72. See Necatigil, op. cit., p. 238.
73. McDonald, 'Cyprus: the UN tries', op. cit., p. 420.
74. Henry Kamm, 'Cypriot Leaders Looking to the US for a Solution', *New York Times*, 3 March 1985.
75. *UN Doc.* S/18102/Add. 1, 11 June 1986.
76. For a full text of the 'Draft Framework Agreement' see appendix 5.
77. *UN Doc.* S/18102/Add. 1, 11 June 1986, Annex V.
78. *UN Doc.* S/18491, 2 December 1986.
79. See *Cyprus Problem, The March 1986 'Draft Framework Agreement' and the Greek Cypriot Side's Attitude Towards It*, Nicosia: Press and Information Office, undated, pp. 3-5.
80. See *Turkish Policy on Cyprus and Efforts to Solve the Cyprus Problem*, Nicosia: Press and Information Office, 1989, pp. 34-5.
81. For a full text of the letter see appendix 6.
82. See UN Doc. S/18102/Add. 1, 11 June 1986, Annex VII.
83. Reuters Despatch, *Cyprus Mail*, 27 April 1986.
84. See UN Doc. S/18102/Add. I, 11 June 1986, Annex V.
85. Quoted in *Turkish Policy on Cyprus*, op. cit., annex 16, p. 119.
86. Ertekun, Necati, *A Memorandum on Efforts to Reach a Negotiated Settlement of the Cyprus Problem and the Constructive Role of the Turkish Cypriot Side to this End* (unpublished), p. 14.
87. Nancy Crawshaw, 'Cyprus: A Failure in Western Diplomacy', *The World Today* vol. 40, no. 2, February 1984, p. 77.
88. *UN Doc.* S/PV 2500, 18 November 1983.
89. See Necatigil, op. cit., pp. 204-5.
90. *House of Commons Debates*, no. 1285, vol. 46, col. 1044.
91. Van Coufoudakis, 'Greek Political Party Attitudes Towards Turkey: 1974-89', in Dimitri Constas, (ed.), *The Greek-Turkish Conflict in the 1990s*, London, Macmillan, 1991, pp. 48-9.
92. Leigh H. Bruce, 'Cyprus. A Last Chance', *Foreign Policy*, no. 58, spring 1985, p. 130.
93. Coufoudakis, op. cit., p. 48.
94. Ibid.
95. Ibid.

96. Crawshaw, op. cit., p. 73.
97. Robert Cutler, 'Soviet Relations with Greece and Turkey: A Systems Perspective' in Dimitri Constas (ed.), op. cit., p. 195.
98. Ibid.
99. Snyder, Jed C., 'Strategic Bias and Southern Flank Security', *Washington Quarterly*, vol. 8, no. 3, summer 1985, p. 135.
100. Coufoudakis, op. cit., pp. 46-7.
101. *New York Times*, 5 July 1980.
102. *The Times*, 17 September 1980.
103. *Turkish Policy on Cyprus*, p. 8.
104. Ibid., p. 9.
105. David Souter, 'An Island Apart: A Review of the Cyprus Problem', *Third World Quarterly* vol. 6, no. 3, July 1984, p. 671.
106. Ibid., p. 673, note 28.
107. Richard, N. Haas, 'Cyprus Moving Beyond Solution', *Washington Quarterly*, vol. 10, no. 2, spring 1987, p. 187.
108. McDonald, op. cit., p. 426.
109. *Cyprus Mail*, 31 March 1984.
110. Snyder, op. cit., p. 132.
111. Bruce, op. cit., p. 131.
112. Crawshaw, op. cit., p. 76.
113. Camp, op. cit., p. 17.
114. See also Bruce, op. cit., p. 129.
115. Quoted by Bruce, op. cit., p. 121.
116. Source does not wish to be identified.
117. Bruce, op. cit., p. 118.
118. Haas, op. cit., p. 183.
119. The Soviet Invasion of Afghanistan and the Iranian Revolution were two events which undermined US influence in the region.
120. See Bruce, op. cit., pp. 118-19.
121. Ibid., p. 115.
122. President Reagan announced on 8 May 1984 his intention to establish a Fund for the cause of a Cyprus solution. The Fund was to be called 'Cyprus Peace and Reconstruction Fund'.
123. Mario Mirdiano, 'Reagan's Letter Generates Cyprus Breakthrough', *The Sunday Times*, 16 December 1984.
124. Quoted in *The New York Times*, 8 July 1984.
125. Haas, op. cit., p. 183.
126. Ibid.
127. See Glen D Camp, 'Cyprus Between the Powers: 1980-1989', *The Cyprus Review*, Nicosia, Intercollege, vol. 1, no. 2, fall 1989, p. 75.
128. Ibid., p. 76.
129. Helen Laipson, 'US Policy Towards Greece and Turkey Since 1974' in Dimitri Constas, op. cit., pp. 169-170.
130. Ibid., p. 171.
131. Ibid., p. 172.
132. Ibid., p. 171.
133. Bruce, op. cit., p. 119.
134. Ibid., p. 133.
135. Ibid., p. 118.
136. Souter, op. cit., p. 673.
137. An instance where the US half-hearted support for the UN was illustrated was when the US abstained on Resolution 550 of the Security Council. For further details see Necatigil, op. cit., p. 222.

138. B. Yegorov, 'Just and Lasting Settlement for Cyprus', *International Affairs*, Moscow, no. 11, November 1984, p. 72.
139. Camp, op. cit., p. 16.
140. The complete text of the Soviet proposals can be found in *Current Digest of the Soviet Press*, vol. 38, no. 3, 19 February 1986, pp. 16-17. Alternatively see *UN Doc.* A/41/96, 21 January 1986.
141. Cutler, op. cit., p. 199.
142. Robert McDonald, 'Cyprus: the gulf widens', *The World Today*, vol. 42, no. 11, November 1986, p. 185.
143. Ibid.

7

AFTER 1986: NEW ACTORS

Since 1986, where we left the last peacemaking effort by the United Nations in Cyprus, there have been various other initiatives – in the late 1980s and up to the middle of 1997 when these pages are being written. So far none has proved successful and therefore one would be justified, at least historically, in viewing the current international effort with the same degree of cynicism as in the past. However, some changes in the 'external' factors may give rise to a certain degree of cautious optimism. We shall try to review the international political climate where the Cyprus problem is concerned since 1986 and how it may have helped to boost the peacemaking efforts of outsiders in the island. The most notable feature of this perhaps is the application by Cyprus in July 1990 to join the European Union and the prospect of its becoming a full member. But first a quick review of the Cyprus problem in its most recent phase.

We shall continue for convenience and clarity to keep to our division of factors to internal and external. Internally both communities followed their convictions as in the past, perhaps with the noticeable difference that the Greek Cypriot leaders have, at least publicly, seemed more willing to compromise than their Turkish Cypriot counterparts. The coming to power of George Vassiliou in 1988 and of the veteran politician, Glafkos Clerides, in 1993 have led to important shifts in the policy of the Cyprus government. However, despite changes in the Turkish Cypriot administration which even led to the Turkish Republican Party sharing power for a while, no such changes have occurred in the position of the Turkish Cypriot leadership on the Cyprus problem. However, on some issues differences have narrowed.

But the most important developments have been external. Some of these relate to the disappearance of bipolarity from the international scene and its replacement by a unipolar system. Others relate to a general feeling of fear and frustration over the Cyprus problem where, although there are casualties – a very small number – from time to time, there is always the danger of tension escalating and causing an armed conflict in the region. The danger has seemed especially great after the Bosnian experience demonstrated the ineptness and inability of the

Europeans to deal with such ethnic crises. But perhaps the most important element in the intensification of peacemaking efforts by the international community is Cyprus's bid to join the EU and the EU's commitment to start negotiations with its government sometime early in 1998, six months after the end of Intergovernmental Talks. It is the latter which has ruffled feathers and alarmed the West.

It has been claimed by some that the most nightmarish scenario for Europe and the West, as well as for Turkey, would be for Cyprus to enter the EU as a full member without a solution to its problem. That would effectively import the Cyprus problem into the EU with all its implications and consequences. Turkey would be in occupation of part of the territory of a member of the European Union, a fact that would dangerously undermine the position of the EU *vis-à-vis* its powerful eastern neighbour and have serious economic and security implications. The United States would also be deeply concerned at having its important NATO ally, and the only Muslim one to boot, disaffected and set at loggerheads with the Europeans. In such an event, Turkey would be in an uncomfortable position and, depending on the government of the day, might feel the need to react negatively. Overall such an eventuality would be troublesome for all concerned.

On the other hand, not to allow Cyprus into the Union also has unpleasant ramifications. Greece has vowed to veto any enlargement of the EU unless and until Cyprus is a full member, and there are no grounds for doubting that it is serious. A Greek veto on this would be diametrically opposed to the plans of the EU advocated in particular by Germany and Britain. This apparent no-win situation for the European Union has meant that every effort is now being made to encourage an early settlement of the conflict. The European Commission is positively engaged in encouraging cooperation from all parties concerned towards a settlement. It has an ambassador based in Nicosia and, though with rather limited resources, is conducting a campaign of information on the benefits of a united Cyprus in the EU, notably among Turkish Cypriots. Hence it can be seen that Cyprus's application to join the EU has led to an intensification of efforts to find a solution, at least by the Europeans, and in that sense it has been a positive move.

The European Union has also been eager to express its determination that no non-member country – meaning Turkey in this instance – can have veto over Cyprus's application. The rationale behind this is that if the absence of a solution is represented as being a permanent obstacle to Cyprus's entry, then Turkey may decide to dig in its heels and not agree to a solution, thereby preventing Cyprus from joining the EU – and by extension prevent a serious rift with the EU from occurring. Not wanting either to upset relations with Turkey or to encounter a Greek veto over its enlargement has led the EU to adopt what the

British call 'constructive ambiguity': Greek Cypriots are encouraged to seek a solution, without which EU accession is unlikely, and Turkey and Turkish Cypriots are also persuaded to be more constructive towards a settlement since EU entry for the Cyprus government (Greek Cypriots) without a solution, though unlikely, is not impossible.

The United States also seems to have taken its peacemaking efforts out of its sluggish bottom gear and is now actively in search of a Cyprus solution. The strongest indication yet is the appointment of Richard Holbrook as the President's Special Representative for the island. Bearing in mind Holbrook's astounding success in Bosnia in the immediate past where everyone else had tried and failed, and the reputation that has inevitably accompanied him ever since, it becomes obvious that this time Americans mean business. But why? What has changed since the 1980s?

First and foremost the absence of the Cold War and the unipolarity of the international system calls, by its very nature, for stability where US foreign policy is concerned, particularly in the eastern Mediterranean region. In the broadest strategic terms it can perhaps be said that in the past the presence of a strong adversary meant that the peace had to be preserved in the region, and now the absence of one requires stability to be maintained for US hegemony to continue. Therefore, a Cyprus solution is advantageous and the lack of one now seems to be a most unnecessary political nuisance.

Secondly, it seems that Turkey may not wish to extend its stay in Cyprus indefinitely. Cyprus has been significant to Turkey, first for reasons of strategy, secondly as a useful negotiating card with Greece, the EU and others, and finally because the Turkish Cypriots are concerned. If a Cyprus solution can guarantee the Turkish Cypriots' political equality, can accommodate Turkey's strategic concerns (for instance demilitarisation of the island and some sort of agreement on those concerns) and finally if it can offer Turkey some concessions over its European ambitions, then Ankara would be very much in favour of a solution. We already know that any solution would entail the first element. We also know that with the huge shifts in the world's geopolitical map, Turkey's strategic and national interests over Cyprus may not be the same as they were in the 1980s. This connects directly with the third element above: firming up Turkey's European vocation and putting its economy in a better shape (with concessions from the EU and the West) may be worth more to Ankara than keeping troops in Cyprus.

However, such an optimistic scenario should be seen against the background of a very difficult history and very disappointing developments. Only in the summer of 1996, as a result of demonstrations organised by motor-cyclists, two Greek Cypriots were killed and a third was shot dead a few days later while in the buffer zone. Although the blame for the killings rests squarely with the authorities in the north, these events obviously do not help the peacemaking process in the island. Experience from other parts of the world also suggests that ethnic strife can be very difficult to manage. A clear example of this exists in Bosnia where, despite the Dayton peace accord and a powerful military presence on the ground, complications occur almost on a regular basis. Northern Ireland is another case where a military presence and external input have both failed to produce an agreement even on paper. The last two examples are particularly significant because both, like Cyprus, are in Europe.

Moreover, the decision by the government of Cyprus to install Russian-made surface-to-air missiles if there is no solution in sight by the middle of 1998 or so – a move that the Cyprus government has stressed is strictly defensive – has angered Turkey. This followed an earlier defence pact between the Greek Cypriots and Greece. These developments may actually produce further inducements for all the parties, external and internal, to search more actively for a solution. But in effect they also raise the stakes and if a further conflict should take place, the consequences may be even more tragic than they were in the past, not only for Cyprus but for others, too. This is particularly so with the nascent peace in the Balkans, where a solution in Cyprus may help the peacekeeping process, while renewed conflict could hinder it.

However, as against all that, the two leaders, President Clerides and Mr Denktash, met in Trout Beck in the United States in July 1997, with further meetings planned for August. It was expected that early in 1998, after the presidential elections in Cyprus, the United Nations would present the two sides with a comprehensive draft paper. Thereafter it would be the political wielding and yielding that would come into play. The input by external players would also be crucial at that time.

It is also noteworthy that Turkey has experienced a change in its domestic political climate. Despite much effort by the Turkish secular establishment to prevent the Islamist Party, Refah, from coming to power, the party actually took office and retained it for over a year. However, in 1997 a coalition of other parties deprived Refah and its coalition partner the True Path Party of their parliamentary majority, and Mesut Yilmaz, leader of the Motherland Party, assumed the premiership. Instability in Turkish domestic political life can mean Turkish indecision over Cyprus. Therefore a period of stability would be helpful should the international momentum for a Cyprus solution continue.

After the death of Andreas Papandreou in Greece, the Greek government appeared more eager to reach a settlement with Turkey over Cyprus. Premier Simitis indicated his willingness to bring the Cyprus saga to an end should Ankara also wish to do so. Despite the skirmishes of the immediate past between the two countries over small Aegean islands, July 1997 witnessed a warming of relations between the two capitals. If there were to be a Cyprus solution in 1998, the background work seemed in July 1997 to be well underway.

So what does all this mean? Are we closer to a Cyprus solution? The answer is inevitably yes, but with the important reminder that we have been there before, maybe even closer to a deal but it failed to materialise (for instance, with the 1977 and the 1979 high-level agreements); and with the proviso that international interest in a solution and the intensity of the search should not diminish in the face of this complex and most volatile political labyrinth. The factors in favour are quite encouraging: President Clinton's stated and active interest in a solution, hence his appointment of Richard Holbrook on the case; Britain's appointment of one of its most senior diplomats, Sir David Hannay, as special envoy for Cyprus (an unprecedented act); the European Union's involvement and the unpleasant consequences for Europe and the West should the *status-quo* continue (the most important element); and finally perhaps a growing maturity on the part of the belligerent parties, both internal and external, and an understanding that the risks associated with the *status quo* may now be greater than the benefits that stem from it.

In the 1990s much change has come about on the international scene. However, we are still, at the time of this writing a long distance from a Cyprus solution but the prospect are definitely better that they were at the beginning of the decade. Premature optimism is (justifiably, of course) the attitude which those professionally engaged in any peace process are obliged to adopt. As someone who has studied and followed the Cyprus problem very closely since the mid-1980s the present writer would warn against such optimistic views just yet. The situation is a most complex and difficult one and many statesmen have tried and failed to solve it in the past. But by no stretch of the imagination is it insoluble. With goodwill and the wielding of sufficient power in the right quarters the Cyprus problem can become a thing of the past. It is to be seen if those elements are present.

August 1997

8
CONCLUSIONS

At the beginning of this study we set out to examine the question of why international peacemaking efforts in Cyprus between 1964 and 1986 failed to bring about a peaceful settlement of the Cyprus problem. The answer must lie in a combination of internal and external factors; intercommunal mistrust and the attitude of outside countries contributed more or less equally to the stalemate.

Internal factor

An example of the deep intercommunal mistrust is the failure of the 1967-74 Intercommunal Talks on the issue of the extent of local government, the Greek Cypriots believing a powerful local government would lead to partition, the Turkish Cypriots fearing a weak local government would result in the domination of the Turkish Cypriots by the Greek Cypriots. This mistrust also contributed to the failure of later efforts.

One of the most notable failures was directly related to the majority-minority issue. International peacemaking in Cyprus failed to change the perceptions of the two sides towards each other: the Greek-Cypriots, though at times the more pliable of the two, continued to view Turkish Cypriots as a minority who should in principle enjoy only minority rights while the Turkish Cypriots continued to perceive Greek Cypriots as the enemy who threatened their lives and livelihood, and therefore aspired to greater autonomy. The two communities' perceptions of each other, and the failure of international peacemaking in changing those perceptions, contributed to the stalemate in Cyprus.

After the invasion in 1974, Turkish Cypriots were eager to translate their superior military position on the ground into political gains at the negotiating table. This became increasingly evident as their stance hardened, making a settlement all the more difficult. In response the Greek Cypriots sought to internationalise the problem further, which only fuelled Turkish Cypriots' irritation.

External Factor

The external factor as regards peacemaking in Cyprus may be seen as consisting of three categories: the United Nations, outside powers and the mother countries.

(a) The United Nations. Throughout the twenty-three years under review, the peacemaking efforts of the international community centred mainly around the United Nations, with the exception of the 1978 joint Initiative by the United States, Britain and Canada. The United Nations' efforts, whether in form of mediation as in the 1964-5 period or the good offices of the Secretary-General, mainly involved the personal involvement of the Secretary-General himself and his personal representative on the island.

Some of the factors necessary for a successful mediation were present in the peacemaking efforts in Cyprus between 1964 and 1986. The process was always informal and flexible, and this suited the parties. It was also confidential and impartial – which was necessary to win the confidence of all sides. If there were leaks to the press they came from the parties themselves and not from the United Nations. There was no sense of finality in the negotiations, so that the two sides were not binding themselves to anything by participating in the intercommunal talks. There was also the prospect of the conflict widening, which heightened the urgency and the importance of a peaceful settlement.

Against these positive factors, there was a lack of coordination between the Security Council and the General Assembly. While the latter impressed upon the former the need to take appropriate measures to implement the contents of the relevant UN resolutions on Cyprus, the Security Council failed to comply. This brings us to another very important point on the role of the UN peacemaking in Cyprus, which is that anything the UN is to do that requires more than the voluntary agreement of the disputants depends on key UN members exerting sufficient and appropriate pressure on them. This never happened in Cyprus in the 1964-86 period. Moreover, there was a divergence of goals between the United Nations and the outside powers. While the UN was mainly trying to introduce a settlement to the disputing parties, the US and other outside powers were concerned to fulfil strategic objectives which were not always compatible. This was especially the case before 1974, when Cyprus posed a more frequent threat to regional peace and security.

The internationalisation of the Cyprus problem by the Greek Cypriots was conducted mainly through the adoption of resolutions at the United Nations which greatly undermined the confidence of the Turkish Cypriots in it. The UN resolutions, whether adopted by the General Assembly or the Security Council, always recognised the government of Cyprus – controlled by Greek Cypriots – as the representative of the state of

Cyprus. They also deplored the Turkish invasion of 1974, called for the withdrawal of foreign troops from Cyprus, and after the UDI by the Turkish-Cypriot leadership in 1983, declared the TRNC illegal. In such ways, the UN afforded the Greek Cypriots moral support and legitimacy for their claims. Naturally, it did not enjoy the same goodwill with the Turkish Cypriots and this adversely affected the process of peacemaking.

Furthermore, Cold War tensions rendered UN resolutions on Cyprus ineffective, noisy barks without biting power. It was unlikely that the Security Council could ever have sanctioned effective measures against any one party in the Cyprus problem, as one of the permanent members of the Council would most probably have vetoed them.

(b) Outside Powers. The Soviet Union throughout the period under review tried to exploit the Cyprus problem for the furtherance of two main objectives: to weaken the south-eastern flank of NATO and to maintain the independence and the non-alignment of Cyprus. However, it had no direct influence on peacemaking in Cyprus.

Britain's efforts tended to fall in with those of the United States; it was careful not to seem partial to either of the parties and was particularly wary of involving itself in a conflict fuelled by intercommunal mistrust. As a guarantor power and the former colonial authority, however, it had the legal right and the political responsibility to strive for a settlement. Ultimately, it acted within the limits of its interests and within the bounds of the possibilities open to it, preferring to act in cooperation with the Americans rather than mount an independent initiative. Canada should also be mentioned in this regard, as it co-sponsored the 1978 Proposal together with Britain and the United States.

The main objectives of the United States in Cyprus emanated from its Cold War policy: to prevent escalation of the conflict in the shape of a Greco-Turkish war and to contain the influence of communism on the island. The failure of its peacemaking efforts stemmed from several factors. One was the lack of a consistent policy: US interest manifested itself only periodically, usually when as in 1964 and 1967, there was the threat of a Greco-Turkish war over Cyprus. Secondly, for most of the period under review, the United States and Makarios never seemed to agree on the outline of a solution, making the formulation of a settlement all the more difficult. Finally, the United States could not afford to put the necessary degree of pressure on Turkey out of fear that such action might result in an improvement in relations between Ankara and Moscow, and a consequent weakening of the south-eastern flank of NATO.

(c) Mother-Countries. However, the most notable failure of peacemaking in Cyprus between 1964 and 1986 concerned the two mother-countries,

Greece and Turkey. Although the international community had, through various United Nations resolutions, diagnosed the internal and the external aspects of the Cyprus problem, it failed to pay sufficient attention to the need to bring Turkey and Greece to the negotiating table. Both of these countries were in a position to exercise great influence over their respective communities in Cyprus, and could therefore be conducive to peacemaking on the island.

Turkey enjoyed a more direct and uninterrupted influence – cultural and political – over Turkish Cypriots than Greece did in relation to the Greek Cypriots. This made the latter less dependent and consequently less compliant: occasionally they acted against the advice of the Greek government as Makarios did in his thirteen constitutional proposals in 1963.

Greece's changing attitude towards Cyprus between 1964 and July 1974 did not help peacemaking efforts on the island; there was continuous tension between the Greek leaders and Makarios, particularly after the military take-over in Greece. While the Greek military regime was keen to reach an agreement with Turkey over Cyprus, Makarios was anxious that no such deals took place, and the inconsistency in the Greek-Greek-Cypriot attitudes made the possibility of a settlement less realistic.

Yet perhaps the most obstructive external factor to a Cyprus settlement between 1974 and 1986 was the unwillingness of Turkey to turn the screws on the Turkish-Cypriot leadership; with its troops in Cyprus, it could have brought about a more favourable response from the Turkish-Cypriot leadership and its unwillingness to do so was the most significant external factor in the failure of international efforts at peacemaking in Cyprus. As we saw, Denktash himself admitted that in the final analysis he would have to go along with the wishes of Ankara, and the uninterrupted support he enjoyed from Turkey between July 1974 and 1986 effectively confirmed its approval of his hard-line stance during negotiations.

Notwithstanding the troublesome nature of the Cyprus problem for Greece and Turkey, the dispute also had its advantages. Both exploited it for their own ends, Turkey looking to Greece for concessions in the Aegean and support for its EC application, and Greece seeking to undermine Turkey's position internationally and to reduce United States aid to that country.

* * * * *

What then are the lessons of this history? What can we learn from it that can help bring about a peaceful settlement to the Cyprus problem?

One safe conclusion is that negotiations alone cannot bridge the wide gap between the two communities, continued after the failure of all peacemaking efforts in the 1964-86 period. Of course there will have to be sacrifices by both communities. Further, political pressure should be applied on the Turkish-Cypriot leadership to soften its tone and be more attuned to the peacemaking efforts of the international community. Without such pressures it is hard to foresee a settlement.

This leads to a second point, which is that the terms of reference of any peacemaker for Cyprus should perhaps be broadened in order to enable definite plans and proposals to be put forward. The UN, in turn, should adopt appropriate procedures to support the peacemaker's proposals and impress on both parties that failure to comply may result in the imposition of harsh measures by the international community. These of course would involve some financial and political costs, and would therefore be adopted only after careful consideration.

The third lesson is that peacekeeping in Cyprus, though it has contributed valuably towards preventing a recurrence of fighting, should perhaps be tied to effective peacemaking measures; in isolation, the peacekeeping force in Cyprus may not be conducive to peacemaking at all. The parties should be made to understand that the failure of peacemaking may in fact lead to the departure of peacekeeping troops from the scene of the conflict. The mere withdrawal in itself, however, would not necessarily lead to an agreement between the disputants. As Alan James put it:

> The general point is that some disputes, of which territorial disputes are the prime instance, are just not soluble by, in effect, threatening to expose the parties to the full consequences of their own intransigence – not least for the reason that it is rare for them to be equally and urgently worried by that prospect. And even if they were, it does not follow that both of them would be willing to settle for something in the nature of half a loaf. Pride and political survival might well stand in the way of that. These comments are illustrated by the particular case of Cyprus. For there is no evidence to suggest that the absence of the UN Force would encourage a more conciliatory frame of mind on either side.[1]

However, the threat of withdrawal could perhaps be made in such a way – and in conjunction with a series of other measures – as to produce the desired result of inducing the parties to move towards a settlement. But in tying peacekeeping to peacemaking it should be borne in mind that the militarily weaker party does not come to a settlement just from fear of being left at the mercy of the stronger; this principle may also hold in other parts of the world where UN peacekeeping operations are being conducted.

Finally, although external pressure in Cyprus is a necessary condition to produce a settlement, it is not sufficient in itself. International factors cannot in themselves effect a resolution. As a matter of practical politics the intercommunal mistrust – the internal factor – should be overcome by mutually agreed measures before external pressures – the external factor – can bring about a settlement. Such confidence-building measures as those referred to in the Security Council Resolution 789 of 24 November 1992 might play an important role in the intercommunal rapprochement. The handing over of Varosha – the modern part of Famagusta – to the UN and the subsequent return of refugees to that city would be one such measure. If it were to be adopted, Greek and Turkish Cypriots might start a process of reintegration in Varosha, overcoming some of their misplaced fears and suspicions of each other.

That the end of the cold war has so far failed to facilitate a Cyprus settlement, perhaps emphasises the significance of intercommunal mistrust in prolonging the dispute. It does not, however, lessen the importance of a united international front in tackling the Cyprus problem, and it is this growing consensus that has enabled the Security Council recently to be more resolute in its approach to the dispute.

Research is still needed to clarify important aspects of the conflict. One obvious topic would be the impact of Greece on the Greek Cypriots concerning international peacemaking efforts. Or alternatively – and perhaps more importantly – the impact of Turkey on the Turkish Cypriot leadership; as Turkey is the principal outside power whose involvement is essential to a solution, it is important to understand the degree of its influence. As yet no thorough and elaborate work has been carried out on these aspects of the Cyprus problem. Such studies, if undertaken, would enable us to understand better the mechanics of Greek/Greek-Cypriot and Turkish/Turkish-Cypriot relations and perhaps enhance the chances of a settlement of the Cyprus problem.

NOTES

1. Alan James, *Peacekeeping in International Politics*, London: Macmillan Academic and Professional Ltd., 1990, p. 236.

APPENDIXES

A

POINTS OF COINCIDENCE AND EQUIDISTANCE OF THE GOBBI INITIATIVE (22 OCTOBER 1981)

POINTS OF EQUIDISTANCE	POINTS OF COINCIDENCE

Part I. General Provisions

1. The Federal Republic of Cyprus shall be an independent, sovereign and non-aligned republic.

2. The territory of the Republic of Cyprus shall compromise the northern and southern provinces and the Federal District.

   (i) The Federal District shall be the seat of the Federal Government.
   (ii) The Northern Province shall be divided into two administrative districts.
   (iii) The Southern Province shall be divided into four administrative districts.

3. Secession, integration or union of the Republic in whole or in part with any other State shall be forbidden, and any act aiming at such union shall be considered a criminal offence punishable by law.

4. The Republic shall have international personality; the federal Government shall exercise sovereignty in respect of all of the territory.

5. The people of the Federal Republic shall compromise the people of the Provinces and the Federal District. There shall be a single citizenship of the Republic of Cyprus regulated by federal law.

6. The Republic of Cyprus shall be demilitarized with the exception of the police forces necessary to maintain law and order in the Provinces and the Federal District.

7. The official languages of the Republic shall be Greek and Turkish. The official working language in federal matters may be English.

8. Each province shall appoint one representative to agree on a neutral federal flag and a national anthem for the Republic. Each province shall create its own flag using, as far as possible, elements of the federal flag. The federal flag shall be flown on federal buildings and federal locations to the exclusion of any other flag.

9. The Federal Government shall observe the holidays of the Republic of Cyprus. Each province shall observe the federal holidays as well as those established locally.

Part II. Fundamental Rights and Liberties

10. Subject to the reinforcement of specific principles in accordance with the Greek Cypriot and Turkish Cypriot proposals (e.g. non-discrimination and equality before the law) and minor drafting changes, Article 6 to 35 of the 1960 Constitution shall apply.

11. Matters relating to education and marriage shall be regulated by the provinces in accordance with the fundamental rights and liberties of the Federal Constitution. Higher education shall be a federal matter.

12. As a transitory provision, two commissions or working groups under the chairmanship of the interlocutors and consisting of six members, three from each province, shall be established to overcome the practical difficulties for the implementation of:

(i) the rights established under Article 13(i) of the 1960 Constitution; and

(ii) the rights established under Article 23 of the 1960 Constitution.

Part III. The Organs of the Federal Government

13. The executive authority of the Republic shall be exercised by a Federal Council composed of six members, one for each administrative district, (2 from the Northern Province and 4 from the Southern Province).

14. The Federal Government shall have the following ministerial portfolios:

(i) Foreign Affairs;

(ii) Defence, Citizenship, Immigration, Emigration, Extradition and Federal Police;

(iii) Justice and Higher Education;

(iv) Co-ordination of International Trade and Tourism, Postal and Tele-communication Services, International Navigation (including authority over ports and airports in connection with international matters);

(v) Federal Finance, Central Bank, Currency, Customs, Weights

15. Members of the Federal Council shall be appointed for five years.

16. The President of the Federal Council shall represent the Republic of Cyprus at home and abroad.

17. The Federal Council of the Republic shall:

(i) Promulgate federal statutes and decisions. Promulgate laws passed by both Chambers;
(ii) Appoint and recall Ambassadors and Envoys;
(iii) Address Letters of Credence and Letters of Recall from foreign diplomatic representatives, issue instruments of ratification and international treaties;
(iv) Confer decorations of the Republic;
(v) Take the necessary measures in the event of an emergency;
(vi) Lay down general principles concerning the internal organization of federal administrative agencies;
(vii) Allocate the federal budget;
(viii) Set the policies of the Federal Government.

18. The Federal Council shall appoint the Federal Attorney General and his Deputy, the Federal Auditor General and his Deputy, the Governor of the Federal Reserve Board and his Deputy, the Federal accountant General and his Deputy. The Deputies shall not be from the same province as their superiors.

19. There shall be an independent Federal Public Service Commission which shall consist of six members, one for each administrative district, to be nominated by the Federal Council. The same ratio of representation, four to two, shall apply in the Council of Ministers and in the Federal Public Service. The federal functions shall be carried out by federal public officers in the Federal District. In other districts federal public officers shall act with the approval of the member of the respective administrative district in the Federal Public Service Commission.

20. The Federal legislative power shall comprise two chambers:

(i) The Chamber of provinces which shall represent the Provinces on an equal basis of ten members each. The Provinces shall assure the proper participation of the administrative districts.

(ii) The Popular Chamber which shall be composed of representatives of the people of Cyprus on a ratio of one member for each 10,000 of the total population.

21. Elections shall be direct and universal. All Cypriot citizens, residents of either of the two provinces, upon attaining the age of 18, shall be qualified to elect.

22. The Federal Supreme Court shall be composed of five members, designated by the Federal Council, two from each Province, and a fifth member who may be a non-Cypriot. The Federal Supreme Court shall have original jurisdiction to hear disputes between the Provinces and shall operate in accordance with the basic provisions of the 1960 Constitution, Articles 153 and 164.

Part IV. Provincial Government

23. The Provinces shall draft their own Constitution in conformity with the Federal Constitution.

24. Each province shall elect by universal suffrage without any kind of discrimination a provincial chamber whose responsibilities shall include approval of the necessary provincial legislation.

25. Each Province shall have no jurisdiction in federal matters. The area of its competence comprehends matters other than those set out in paragraph 14.

26. Each Province shall establish its own administration of justice and will control the provincial police.

Part V. Transitional Provisions

27. The Province shall establish a Joint Board of Claims to deal with compensation claims arising from the establishment of the Republic. The Federal Supreme Court shall act as a Court of Appeal for the decisions of the Board. The Federal Supreme Court shall establish a summary proceeding to deal expeditiously with these claims.

28. A Fund for Development of the Northern Province shall be established with a view to achieving an economic equilibrium between the two Provinces. The Federal Government shall contribute to this Fund. Foreign Governments and international organizations shall be invited to contribute to the Fund.

29. A Federal Real Estate Bank shall be established to provide credit and economic assistance to displaced persons for the purpose of their permanent settlement.

B

GENERAL ASSEMBLY RESOLUTION 37/253 (1983)

The UN General Assembly adopted resolution 37/253 on Cyprus on May 13, 1983. The vote on the resolution was 103 in favour and 5 against with 20 abstentions. The votes against the resolution were cast by Bangladesh, Malaysia, Pakistan, Somalia and Turkey.

Following is the text of the resolution:

The General Assembly,

Having considered the question of Cyprus,

Recalling its resolution 3212 (XXIX) of 1 November 1974 and its subsequent resolutions on the question of Cyprus,

Recalling the high-level agreements of 12 February 1977 and 19 May 1979,

Reaffirming the principle of the inadmissibility of occupation and acquisition of territories by force,

Greatly concerned at the prolongation of the Cyprus crisis, which poses a serious threat to international peace and security,

Deeply regretting that the resolutions of the United Nations on Cyprus have not yet been implemented,

Recalling the idea of holding an international conference on Cyprus,

Deploring the fact part of the territory of the Republic of Cyprus is still occupied by foreign forces,

Deploring the lack of progress in the intercommunal talks,

Deploring all unilateral actions that change the demographic structure of Cyprus or promote faits accomplis,

Reaffirming the need to settle the question of Cyprus without further delay by peaceful means in accordance with the provisions of the Charter of the United Nations and the relevant United Nations resolutions:

1. *Reiterates* its full support for the sovereignty, independence, territorial integrity, unity and non-alignment of the Republic of Cyprus and calls once again for the cessation of all foreign interference in its affairs;

2. *Affirms* the right of the Republic of Cyprus and its people to full and effective sovereignty and control over the entire territory of Cyprus and its natural and other resources and calls upon all states to support and help the Government of the Republic of Cyprus to exercise these rights;

3. *Condemns* any act which tends to undermine the full and effective exercise of the above-mentioned rights, including the unlawful issue of titles of ownership of property;
4. *Welcomes* the proposal for total demilitarization made by the President of the Republic of Cyprus;
5. *Express its support* for the high-level agreements of 12 February 1977 and 19 May 1979 and all the provisions thereof;
6. *Demands* the immediate and effective implementation of resolution 3212 (XXIX), unanimously adopted by the General assembly and endorsed by the Security Council in its resolution 365 (1974) of 13 December 1974, and of the subsequent resolutions of the Assembly and the Council on Cyprus which provide the valid and essential basis for the solution of the problem of Cyprus;
7. *Considers* the withdrawal of all occupation forces from the Republic of Cyprus as an essential basis for an speedy and mutually acceptable solution of the Cyprus problem;
8. *Demands* the immediate withdrawal of all occupation forces from the Republic of Cyprus;
9. *Commends* the intensification of the efforts made by the Secretary-General, while noting with concern the lack of progress in the intercommunal talks;
10. *Calls* for meaningful, result-oriented, constructive and substantive negotiations between the representatives of the two communities, under the auspices of the Secretary-General, to be conducted freely and on an equal footing, on the basis of relevant United Nations resolutions and the high-level agreements, with a view to reaching as early as possible a mutually acceptable agreement based on the fundamental and legitimate rights of the two communities;
11. *Calls* for respect of the human rights and fundamental freedoms of all Cypriots, including the freedom of movement, the freedom of settlement and the right to property and the instituting of urgent measures for the voluntary return of the refugees to their homes in safety;
12. *Considers* that the *de facto* situation created by the force of arms should not be allowed to influence or in any way affect the solution of the problem of Cyprus;
13. *Calls upon* the parties concerned to refrain from any unilateral action which might adversely affect the prospects of a just and lasting solution of the problem of Cyprus by peaceful means and to cooperate fully with the Secretary-General in the performance of his task under the relevant resolutions of the General Assembly and the Security Council as well as with the United Nations Peace-Keeping Force in Cyprus;
14. *Calls upon* the parties concerned to refrain from any action which violates or is designed to violate the independence, unity, sovereignty and territorial integrity of the Republic of Cyprus;

15. *Reiterates* its recommendation that the Security Council should examine the question of implementation, within a specified time-frame, of its relevant resolutions and consider and adopt thereafter, if necessary, all appropriate and practical measures under the Charter of the United Nations for ensuring the speedy and effective implementation of the resolutions of the United Nations on Cyprus;
16. *Welcomes* the intention of the Secretary-General, as expressed in his report (Doc. A/37/805 of 6/5/1983), to pursue a renewed personal involvement in the quest for a solution of the Cyprus problem and, in view of this, requests the Secretary-General to undertake such actions or initiatives as he may consider appropriate within the framework of the mission of good offices entrusted to him by the Security Council for promoting a just and lasting solution of the problem and to report to the General Assembly at its thirty-eighth session on the results of his efforts;
17. *Decides* to include in the provisional agenda of its thirty-eighth session the item entitled 'Question of Cyprus' and requests the Secretary-General to follow up the implementation of the present resolution and to report on all its aspects to the General Assembly at that session.

Separate vote on Paragraph 8

Separate votes were taken on operative Paragraph 8 which asks for the withdrawal of all occupation forces from the Republic of Cyprus.
89 countries voted in favour, 5 against and 27 abstained.

Separate vote on Paragraph 15

Separate votes were also taken on operative Paragraph 15 which recommends that the Security Council should examine the question of implementation, within a specified time-frame, of its relevant resolutions and to consider and adopt practical measures for the implementation of U.N. resolutions on Cyprus.
86 countries voted in favour, 8 against and 25 abstained.

C

ITEM PUBLISHED IN THE *CYPRUS MAIL*, 18 AUGUST 1983

Aide-Mémoire Text

The following is the text of the 'Aide-Mémoire' delivered to the Greek and Turkish Cypriot sides earlier this month by the UN Special Representative Hugo Gobbi containing the views of the Secretary-General Pérez de Cuéllar for the resumption of meaningful talks with restricted goals in the first instance.

No official text has been released but extracts have appeared in Turkish papers and *Phileleftheros* yesterday said that after the leaks there was no reason why the text should not be made known.

This note, a two-page document, variously described as 'Aide-Memoire' or 'Non-Paper', as published in *Phileleftheros* says:

1. The Secretary-General has undertaken a personal effort to lend fresh impetus to the intercommunal negotiating process, within the framework of the mission of Good Offices entrusted to him by the Security Council. This effort is intended to follow up the work done during the current round of the Intercommunal Talks, which remain the formal negotiating forum.

As part of this effort, the Secretary-General will be sounding out the parties concerned on ways and means of furthering the negotiating process.

2. As a first step, the Secretary-General wishes to know whether the parties concerned would find it appropriate to pursue the negotiations within the frame of certain 'indicators'.

Three such indicators, covering major unresolved issues in the 'Evaluation' paper (Waldheim's) are outlined below. If this approach proves acceptable, further suggested indicators will be forthcoming in due course.

3. (a) The elected head of the Southern Province will be appointed President of the Federal Republic and the elected head of the Northern Province, Vice President. Members of the two provinces all be represented in the Federal Executive in a proportion of 60/40 (GkCyp/TkCyp) respectively.

(or) The elected heads of the Southern and Northern Provinces will be appointed Head of State and Government respectively on a rotation basis. Members of the Provinces shall be represented in the Federal Executive in the proportion of 70 per cent (GkCyp) and 30 per cent (TkCyp).

(b) Legislative:

The Federal Republic shall have a bicameral system: the Lower Chamber will have its members elected according to the principle of proportional representation; both Provinces shall be equally represented in the Upper Chamber.

(or) The Federal Republic shall have a bicameral system. The Lower Chamber shall be composed of members elected by the Turkish Cypriot community in the proportion of 30 per cent and by the Greek Cypriot community in the proportion of 70 per cent. Both Provinces shall be equally represented in the Upper Chamber.

(c) Territory

The territory of the Southern Province shall cover 77 per cent of the territory of the republic, that of the Northe*rn Province 23 per cent of it.

(or) The territory of the Southern Province will cover 70 per cent of the territory of the republic, that of the Northern Province 30 per cent of it.

4. If the Parties agree to the above 'indicators' they will be transmitted by the Special Representative of the Secretary-General to the Interlocutors at the Intercommunal Talks, who will proceed to negotiate within the limits defined by the said indicators. The same procedure will be used in relation to additional indicators.

5. The Secretary-General would appreciate it if he could be informed of the reactions of the Parties by 15 September 1983. He considers this sounding to have been made in utmost confidentiality and requests that all possible measures be taken to maintain its confidential and strictly informal character.

D

SECURITY COUNCIL RESOLUTION 541 (1983)

The UN Security Council adopted on 18 November 1983 Resolution 541 (1983) by 13 votes in favour, one against (Pakistan) and one abstention (Jordan).

The adopted text reads as follows:

The Security Council,

Having heard the statement of the Foreign Minister of the Government of the Republic of Cyprus,

Concerned at the Declaration by the Turkish Cypriot authorities issued on 15 November 1983 which purports to create an independent state in northern Cyprus,

Considering that this Declaration is incompatible with the 1960 Treaty concerning the establishment of the Republic of Cyprus and the 1960 Treaty of Guarantee,

Considering therefore that the attempt to create a 'Turkish Republic of Northern Cyprus' is invalid, and will contribute to a worsening of the situation in Cyprus,

Reaffirming its resolutions 365 (1974) and 367 (1975),

Aware of the need for a solution of the Cyprus problem, based on the mission of good offices undertaken by the Secretary-General,

Affirming its continuing support for the United Nations Peace-Keeping Force in Cyprus,

Taking note of the Secretary-General's statement of 17 November 1983:

1. *Deplores* the Declaration of the Turkish Cypriot authorities of the purported secession of part of the Republic of Cyprus;
2. *Considers* the Declaration referred to above as legally invalid and calls for its withdrawal;
3. *Calls* for the urgent and effective implementation of its resolutions 365 (1974) and 367 (1975);
4. *Requests* the Secretary-General to pursue his mission of good offices in order to achieve the earliest possible progress towards a just and lasting settlement in Cyprus;
5. *Calls upon* the parties to cooperate fully with the Secretary-General in his mission of good offices;

6. *Calls upon* all states to respect the sovereignty, independence, territorial integrity and non-alignment of the Republic of Cyprus;
7. *Calls upon* all states not to recognize any Cypriot state other than the Republic of Cyprus;
8. *Calls upon* all states and the two communities in Cyprus to refrain from any action which might exacerbate the situation;
9. *Requests* the Secretary-General to keep the Security Council fully informed.

E

DRAFT FRAMEWORK AGREEMENT ON CYPRUS, 29 MARCH 1986

Recognising with satisfaction that the initiative of the Secretary-General, which bore in mind the relevant United Nations resolutions and which began in August 1984 in Vienna and continued through the high-level proximity talks from September to December 1984 and the joint high-level meeting of January 1985 held in New York, has now resulted in an important step towards a just and lasting settlement of the Cyprus problem;

The parties agree on the following matters which are to be viewed as an integrated whole:

1.1 The Parties:

(a) Recommit themselves to the high-level agreements of 1977 and 1979;

(b) Indicate their determination to proceed, at the date referred to in paragraph 15.1 below, to the establishment of a Federal Republic that will be independent and non-aligned, bi-communal as regards the federal constitutional aspect and bi-zonal as regards the territorial aspect;

(c) Reaffirm their acceptance of those introductory constitutional provisions that were agreed upon at the intercommunal talks in 1981-82;

(i) The Federal Republic of Cyprus shall have international personality. The federal government shall exercise sovereignty in respect of all of the territory. The attributes of international personality shall be exercised by the federal government in accordance with the federal constitution. The provinces or federated states may act in their areas of competence in accordance with the federal constitution and in a manner that would not duplicate the powers and functions of the federal government as defined in the federal constitution.

(ii) The people of the Federal Republic shall comprise the Greek Cypriot community and the Turkish Cypriot community. There shall be a single citizenship of the Federal Republic of Cyprus regulated by federal law.

(iii) The territory of the Federal Republic shall comprise the two provinces or federated states.

(iv) The official languages of the Federal Republic shall be Greek and Turkish. The English language may also be used.

(v) The Federal Republic shall have a neutral flag and anthem to be agreed. Each province or federated state may have its own flag using mainly elements of the federal flag. The federal flag shall be flown on federal buildings and federal locations to the exclusion of any other flag.

(vi) The federal government shall observe the holidays of the Federal Republic. Each province or federated state shall observe the federal holidays as well as those established by it.

(vii) The parties reaffirm all other points that were agreed upon during the course of the intercommunal talks as contained in the 'revision' dated 18 May 1982 concerning general provisions, Part I, fundamental rights and liberties, Part II, as well as Parts III and IV.

2.1 The powers and functions to be vested in the federal government of the Federal Republic shall comprise:

(a) Foreign affairs.

(b) Federal financial affairs (including federal budget, taxation, customs and excise duties).

(c) Monetary and banking affairs.

(d) Federal economic affairs (including trade and tourism).

(e) Posts and telecommunications.

(f) International transport.

(g) Natural resources (including water supply, environment).

(h) Federal health and veterinary affairs.

(i) Standard setting: weights and measures, patents, trademarks, copyrights.

(j) Federal judiciary.

(k) Appointment of federal officers.

(l) Defence (to be discussed also in connection with the treaties of guarantee and of alliance); security (as it pertains to federal responsibility).

2.2 Additional powers and functions may be vested in the federal government by common agreement of both sides. Accordingly, the residual powers shall rest with the provinces or federated states. Federal legislation may be executed either by authorities of the federal government or by way of coordination between the competent authorities of the federal government and of the two provinces or federated states.

3.1 The legislature of the Federal Republic will be composed of two chambers: a lower chamber with a 70-30 Greek Cypriot and Turkish Cypriot representation, and an upper chamber with a 50-50 representation. Federal legislation will be enacted with regard to the matters of federal competence as referred to in paragraph 2.1 above. The adoption of legislation on major matters, as for instance on ten of the twelve functions referred to in paragraph 2.1 above, will require separate majorities in both chambers. The adoption of legislation on other matters will require majorities of the membership in each chamber.

3.2 Appropriate constitutional safeguards and deadlock resolving machinery including special provisions to facilitate action on matters necessary for the continued functioning of the federal government (e.g. on budgetary questions) will be incorporated in the federal constitution. In case of deadlock in the legislature, the proposed legislation may be submitted in the first instance to a conciliation committee of the legislature composed of three Greek Cypriots and two Turkish Cypriots, whose decision will be taken on the basis of majority vote including at least one Turkish Cypriot. If the deadlock persists, the president and vice-president of the Federal Republic will, upon request, appoint on an *ad hoc* basis one persons each, selected for their knowledge of the subject involved, who, with the assistance of experts as needed, including from outside the Federal Republic of Cyprus, will advise the legislature on ways the deadlock could be resolved. The matter may also be submitted to a referendum among the population of the community which opposed the draft legislation. Legislation adopted by the legislature may be taken to the Constitutional Court for ruling as to whether it violates the constitution or is discriminatory against either community.

4.1 The Federal Republic will have a presidential system of government. The president and the vice-president will symbolise the unity of the country and the equal political status of the two communities. In addition, the executive will reflect the functional requirements of an effective federal government.

4.2 The president will be a Greek Cypriot and the vice-president will be a Turkish Cypriot. The president and the vice-president will, separately or conjointly, have the right to veto any law or decision of the legislature and the Council of Ministers in areas to be agreed upon, it being understood that the scope will exceed that covered by the 1960 constitution. The president and the vice-president will have the right, separately or conjointly, to return any law or decision of the legislature or any decision of the Council of Ministers for reconsideration.

4.3 The Council of Ministers will be composed of Greek Cypriot and Turkish Cypriot ministers on a 7 to 3 ratio. One major ministry will be headed by a Turkish Cypriot, it being understood that the parties agree to discuss that the Minister for Foreign Affairs will be a Turkish Cypriot. The Council of Ministers will take decisions by weighted voting, that is a simple majority including at least one Turkish Cypriot minister. It is understood that the parties agree to discuss that weighted voting will apply to all matters of special concern to the Turkish Cypriot community to be agreed upon.

4.4 Appropriate constitutional safeguards and deadlock resolving machinery related to decisions by the Council of Ministers, including special provisions to facilitate action on matters necessary for the continued functioning of the federal government, will be incorporated in the federal constitution. In case of deadlock, the president and vice-president of the Federal Republic will, upon request, appoint on an *ad hoc* basis one person each, selected for their knowledge of the subject involved, who, with the assistance of experts as needed, including from outside the Federal Republic of Cyprus, will advise the Council of Ministers on ways the deadlock could be resolved. The matter may also be submitted to a referendum among the population of the community which opposed the draft decision. A decision by the Council of Ministers may be taken to the Constitutional Court for ruling as to whether it violates the constitution or is discriminatory against either community.

5.1 The Constitutional Court, when ruling on disputes relating to the distribution of powers and functions between the federal government and the provinces or federated states and on such other matters as may be assigned to it by the parties in accordance with the federal constitution, will be composed of one Greek Cypriot, one Turkish Cypriot and one non-Cypriot voting member.

6.1 As regards freedom of movement, freedom of settlement and right to property, a working group will discuss the exercise of these rights, including time-frames, practical regulations and possible compensation arrangements, taking into account guideline 3 of the 1977 agreement.

7.1 Territorial adjustments, in addition to the areas already referred to in the 5 August 1981 Turkish Cypriot proposals, will be agreed upon. These territorial adjustments will result in the Turkish Cypriot province or federated state comprising in the order of 29 plus per cent of the territory of the Federal Republic. It is understood that when discussing the actual territorial adjustments the two sides will have in mind the 1977 high-level agreement including 'certain practical difficulties which may arise for the Turkish Cypriot community' and the questions related to resettlement. Both sides agree to suggest special status areas adjacent to each other for the purpose of enhancing trust between the sides. These areas will remain under their respective civilian jurisdictions.

8.1 A timetable for the withdrawal of non-Cypriot military troops and elements, as well as adequate guarantees, will be agreed upon prior to the establishment of a transitional federal government. In the meantime, military deconfrontation measures will be pursued by both sides, using the good offices and assistance of UNFICYP.

8.2 The two sides undertake to discuss these issues in good faith and to consider each other's concerns on them.

9.1 A Fund for Development of the Turkish Cypriot province or federated state shall be established with a view to achieving an economic equilibrium between the two provinces or federated states. A fund will also be established to facilitate the resettlement of the Greek Cypriot displaced persons, and for the Turkish Cypriots displaced as a consequence of the implementation of paragraph 7.1. The federal government shall contribute to these funds. Foreign governments and international organisations shall be invited to contribute to the funds.

10.1 The Varosha area and the six additional areas delineated in the Turkish Cypriot map of 5 August 1981 will be placed under United Nations interim administration as part of the UNFICYP buffer zone for resettlement by....

11.1 Both parties agree not to take any action tending to prejudice the process outlined in this agreement, both on the international scene and internally.

12.1 The Nicosia international airport will be reopened under interim United Nations administration with free access from both sides. The United Nations will conclude the arrangements to that effect by....

13.1 Adequate machinery for considering allegations of non-implementation of confidence-building measures will be agreed upon. The Secretary-General will make appropriate recommendations to both sides in this regard.

14.1 The parties to agree to establish working groups to work out the detailed agreements on the matters referred to in this agreement, whose elements are inter-related and constitute an integrated whole. The working groups will carry out their work under the direction of joint high-level meetings. These joint high-level meetings will take place every three to four months, on the basis of an agenda prepared by the Secretary-General, to discuss the issues which remain to be negotiated under this agreement, to review the work and provide guidance to the working groups. The joint high-level meetings will be convened by the Secretary-General after adequate preparation.

14.2 Each working group will be composed of delegations from the two sides and will be chaired by a representative of the Secretary-General. The working groups will begin their meetings at the United Nations premises in Nicosia on.... Each working group will prepare a programme of work and will submit it for approval and guidance to the joint high-level meeting which will take place at the United Nations premises in Nicosia on....

14.3 The representative of the Secretary-General chairing each working group will every three months prepare an assessment of the progress made by the working group, which will be presented to the next joint high-level meeting together with the views of the Secretary-General.

15.1 The parties agree that, the required working groups having completed their work and having obtained the approval of the two sides, the transitional federal government of the Federal Republic of Cyprus will be set up on....

16.1 The Secretary-General will remain at the disposal of the parties to assist in the elaboration of this agreement, and, if required, in its interpretation.

F

LETTER OF PRESIDENT KYPRIANOU TO THE U.N. SECRETARY-GENERAL, 20 APRIL 1986

Dear Mr Secretary-General,

I acknowledge receipt of your letter of 29 March, 1986 with which you enclosed the document entitled 'Draft Framework Agreement'.

I should like to assure you that we are committed to a just and lasting solution of the Cyprus problem as a matter of urgency. It is precisely because of that commitment that we believe that, before the Greek Cypriot side expresses its views on the contents of the 'Draft Framework Agreement' you have presented, it is necessary that there be agreement on the basic issues of the Cyprus problem as a matter of priority.

For this reason I request you to adopt one of two alternative procedures:

I. To convene an International Conference in respect of the international aspects of the Cyprus problem, namely,

1. Withdrawal of the Turkish forces of occupation and settlers; and
2. Effective international guarantees.

II. In the event that the holding of such an International Conference proves impossible, to convene a High Level Meeting to deal with the following matters, namely,

1. Withdrawal of the Turkish forces of occupation and settlers;
2. Effective international guarantees; and
3. Application of the three freedoms, that is freedom of movement, freedom of settlement and the right to property.

These issues should be resolved in conformity with the UN Charter and Security Council and General Assembly Resolutions on Cyprus, including Security Council Resolutions 541 and 550.

I am anxious that your mission of good offices should succeed and I consider that adoption of one of these two procedures is the best way to ensure that rapid progress is made to a just and lasting solution of the Cyprus problem.

Please accept, Your Excellency, the assurances of my highest consideration.

SPYROS KYPRIANOU
President of the Republic of Cyprus

G

SECURITY COUNCIL RESOLUTIONS 186, 353 AND 357 AND GENERAL ASSEMBLY RESOLUTION 3212 (XXIX)

RESOLUTION 186 (1964)

adopted by the Security Council, 4 March 1964

The Security Council,

Noting that the present situation with regard to Cyprus is likely to threaten international peace and security and may further deteriorate unless additional measures are promptly taken to maintain peace and to seek out a durable solution,

Considering the positions taken by the parties in relation to the Treaties signed at Nicosia on 16 August 1960,

Having in mind the relevant provisions of the Charter of the United Nations and its Article 2, paragraph 4, which reads: 'All Members shall refrain in their international relations from the threat or use of force against the territorial integrity or political independence of any State, or in any other manner inconsistent with the purposes of the United Nations',

1. *Calls upon* all Member States, in conformity with their obligations under the charter of the United Nations, to refrain from any action or threat of action to worsen the situation in the sovereign Republic of Cyprus, or to endanger international peace;

2. *Asks* the Government of Cyprus, which has the responsibility for the maintenance and restoration of law and order, to take all additional measures necessary to stop violence and bloodshed in Cyprus;

3. *Calls upon* the communities in Cyprus and their leaders to act with the utmost restraint;

4. *Recommends* the creation, with the consent of the Government of Cyprus, of a United Nations Peace-Keeping Force in Cyprus. The composition and size of the Force shall be established by the Secretary-General, in consultation with the Governments of Cyprus, Greece, Turkey and the United Kingdom. The commander of the Force shall be appointed by the Secretary-General and report to him. The Secretary-General,

who shall keep the Governments providing the Force fully informed, shall report periodically to the Security Council on its operation;
5. *Recommends* that the function of the Force should be in the interest of preserving international peace and security, to use its best efforts to prevent a recurrence of fighting and, as necessary, to contribute to the maintenance and restoration of law and order and a return to normal conditions;
6. *Recommends* that the stationing of the Force shall be for a period of three months, all costs pertaining to it being met, in a manner to be agreed upon by them, by the Governments providing the contingents and by the Government of Cyprus. The Secretary-General may also accept voluntary contributions for that purpose;
7. *Recommends further* that the Secretary-General designate, in agreement with the Government of Cyprus and the Governments of Greece, Turkey and United Kingdom a mediator who shall use his best endeavours with the representatives of the communities and also with the aforesaid four Governments, for the purpose of promoting a peaceful solution and an agreed settlement of the problem confronting Cyprus, in accordance with the Charter of the United Nations, having in mind the well-being of the people of Cyprus as a whole and the preservation of international peace and security. The mediator shall report periodically to the Secretary General on his efforts;
8. *Requests* the Secretary-General to provide, from funds of the United Nations, as appropriate, for the remuneration and expenses of the mediation and his staff.

Adopted unanimously at the 1102nd meeting.

RESOLUTION 353 (1974)

adopted by the Security Council, 20 July 1974

The Security Council,

Having considered the report of the Secretary-General at its 1779th meeting about the recent developments in Cyprus,
Having heard the statement made by the President of the Republic of Cyprus and the statements by the representatives of Cyprus, Turkey, Greece and other Member States,
Having considered at its present meeting further developments in the island,
Deeply deploring the outbreak of violence and continuing bloodshed,
Gravely concerned about the situation which led to a serious threat to

international peace and security, and which created a most explosive situation in the whole Eastern Mediterranean area,

Equally concerned about the necessity to restore the constitutional structure of the Republic of Cyprus, established and guaranteed by international agreement,

Recalling, its resolution 186 (1964) of 4 March 1964 and its subsequent resolutions on this matter,

Conscious of this primary responsibility for the maintenance of international peace and security in accordance with Article 24 of the Charter of the United Nations,

1. *Calls upon* all States to respect the sovereignty, independence and territorial integrity of Cyprus;
2. *Calls upon* all parties to the present fighting as a first step to cease all firing and requests all States to exercise the utmost restraint and to refrain from any action which might further aggravate the situation;
3. *Demands* an immediate end to foreign military intervention in the Republic of Cyprus that is in contravention of paragraph 1 above;
4. *Requests* the withdrawal without delay from the Republic of Cyprus of foreign military personnel present otherwise than under the authority of international agreements, including those whose withdrawal was requested by the President of the Republic of Cyprus, Archbishop Makarios, in his letter of 2 July 1974;
5. *Calls upon* Greece, Turkey and the United Kingdom of Great Britain and Northern Ireland to enter into negotiation without delay for the restoration of peace in the area and constitutional government in Cyprus and to keep the Secretary-General informed;
6. *Calls upon* all parties to cooperate fully with the United Nations Peace-Keeping Force in Cyprus to enable it to carry out its mandate;
7. *Decides* to keep the situation under constant review and asks the Secretary-General to report as appropriate with a view to adopting further measures in order to ensure that peaceful conditions are restored as soon as possible.

Adopted unanimously at the 1781st meeting.

RESOLUTION 357 (1974)

adopted by the Security Council on 14 August 1974

The Security Council,

Recalling its resolutions 353 (1974) of 20 July 1974, 354 (1974) of 23 July 1974 and 355 (1974) of 1 August 1974,

Deeply deploring the resumption of fighting in Cyprus contrary to the provisions of its resolution 353 (1974),
1. *Reaffirms* its resolution 353 (1974) in all its provisions and calls upon the parties concerned to implement those provisions without delay;
2. *Demands* that all parties to the present fighting cease all firing and military action forthwith;
3. *Calls for* the resumption of negotiations without delay for the restoration of peace in the area and constitutional government in Cyprus in accordance with resolution 353 (1974);
4. *Decides* to remain seized of the situation and on instant call to meet as necessary to consider what more effective measures may be required if the cease-fire is not respected.

Adopted unanimously at the 1792nd meeting.

RESOLUTION 3212 (XXIX)

The General Assembly adopted on the evening of 1st November, 1974, resolution 3212 (XXIX) by 117 votes in favour, none against and no abstentions.

The resolution reads as follows:

The General Assembly,

Having considered the question of Cyprus,
Gravely concerned about the continuation of the Cyprus crisis, which constitutes a threat to international peace and security,
Mindful of the need to solve this crisis without delay by peaceful means, in accordance with the purposes and principles of the United Nations,
Having heard the statements in the debate and taking note of the Report of the Special Political Committee on the Question of Cyprus,
1. *Calls upon* all states to respect the sovereignty, independence, territorial integrity and non-alignment of the Republic of Cyprus and to refrain from all acts and interventions directed against it;
2. *Urges* the speedy withdrawal of all foreign armed forces and foreign military presence and personnel from the Republic of Cyprus and the cessation of all foreign interference in its affairs;
3. *Considers* that the constitutional system of the Republic of Cyprus concerns the Greek-Cypriot and Turkish-Cypriot communities;
4. *Commends* the contacts and negotiations taking place on an equal footing, with the good offices of the Secretary-General between the representatives of the two communities, and calls for their continuation

with a view to reaching freely a mutually acceptable political settlement, based on their fundamental and legitimate rights;

5. *Considers* that all the refugees should return to their homes in safety and calls upon the parties concerned to undertake urgent measures to that end;

6. *Expresses* the hope that, if necessary, further efforts including negotiations can take place, within the framework of the United Nations, for the purpose of implementing the provisions of the present resolution, thus ensuring to the Republic of Cyprus its fundamental right to independence, sovereignty and territorial integrity;

7. *Requests* the Secretary-General to continue to provide United Nations humanitarian assistance to all parts of the population of Cyprus and calls upon all states to contribute to that effort;

8. *Calls upon* all parties to continue to cooperate fully with the United Nations Peace-Keeping Force in Cyprus, which may be strengthened if necessary;

9. *Requests* the Secretary-General to continue to lend his good offices to the parties concerned;

10. *Further requests* the Secretary-General to bring the present resolution to the attention of the Security Council.

BIBLIOGRAPHY

PRIMARY SOURCES

OFFICIAL DOCUMENTS AND PRIVATE MEMORANDA

The United Nations

Charter of the United Nations.
Galo Plaza Report, United Nations Security Council Official Records, Supplement January-June 1965, S/6253, 26 March 1965
Reports of the Secretary-General on the United Nations' Operation in Cyprus, March 1964 to November 1967.
Reports of the Secretary-General on his mission of good offices in Cyprus, 1967 to 1986.
Repertory of Practice of United Nations Organs, vol. 1, paras. 221-229; Supplement No. 1, vol. 1, paras. 152-155; Supplement No. 3, Vol. 1.

Security Council Resolutions

186, 4 March 1964
187, 13 March 1964
192, 20 June 1964
193, 9 August 1964
194, 25 September 1964
198, 18 December 1964
201, 19 March 1965
206, 15 June 1965
207, 10 August 1965
219, 17 December 1965
220, 16 March 1966
222, 16 June 1966
231, 15 December 1966
238, 19 June 1967
244, 22 December 1967
247, 18 March 1968
254, 18 June 1968
261, 10 December 1968
266, 10 June 1969
274, 11 December 1969
281, 9 June 1970
291, 10 December 1970
293, 26 May 1971
305, 13 December 1971

315, 15 June 1972
324, 12 December 1972
334, 15 June 1973
343, 14 December 1973
349, 29 May 1974
353, 20 July 1974
354, 23 July 1974
355, 1 August 1974
357, 14 August 1974
358, 15 August 1974
359, 15 August 1974
360, 16 August 1974
361, 30 August 1974
364, 13 December 1974
365, 13 December 1974
367, 12 March 1975
370, 13 June 1975
383, 13 December 1975
391, 15 June 1976
401, 14 December 1976
410, 15 June 1977
414, 15 September 1977
422, 15 December 1977
430, 16 June 1978
440, 27 November 1978
443, 14 December 1978
451, 15 June 1979
458, 14 December 1979
472, 13 June 1980
482, 1 December 1980
488, 4 June 1981
495, 14 December 1981
510, 15 June 1982
526, 14 December 1982
534, 15 June 1983
541, 18 November 1983
544, 15 December 1983
550, 11 May 1984
553, 15 June 1984
559, 15 December 1984
565, 15 June 1985
578, 12 December 1985
585, 13 June 1986
593, 11 December 1986

Security Council Debates

S/PV/532, 21 February 1951
S/PV/763, 23 January 1959

S/PV 1779, 16 July 1974
S/PV 1780, 19 July 1974
S/PV 1781, 20 July 1974
S/PV 1782, 22 July 1974
S/PV 1783, 23 July 1974
S/PV 1785, 27 July 1974
S/PV 1788, 31 July 1974
S/PV 1792, 14 August 1974
S/PV 1793, 15 August 1974
S/PV 1794, 16 August 1974
S/PV 1817, 27 February 1975
S/PV 1973, 19 November 1976
S/PV 2012, 15 June 1977
S/PV 2013, 16 June 1977
S/PV 2500, 18 November 1983
S/PV 2565, 14 December 1984

Security Council Documents

S/597, 3 November 1947
S/651, 17 January 1948
S/1791, 15 September 1950
S/2017/Rev. 1, 30 March 1951
S/2967, 27 March 1953
S/3821, 29 April 1957
S/5169, 25 May 1962
S/5593/Add. 3, 26 March 1964
S/5950, 10 September 1964
S/6228, 11 March 1965
S/6253 and Corr. 1, 26 March 1965
S/6569, 29 July 1965
S/66/47, 1 September 1965
S/6683, 16 September 1965
S/7191, 10 March 1966
S/7221, 24 March 1966
S/7231, 1 April 1966
S/8248, 16 November 1967
S/10401, 18 October 1971, Chapter V
S/10664, 26 May 1972
S/11137, 1 December 1973
S/11353, Add. 20, 21 July 1974
S/11398, 1 August 1974
S/11433, 10 August 1974
S/11624, 18 February, 1975, Annex B
S/11659, 21 March 1975
S/11717, 9 June 1975
S/11789, 5 August 1975
S/11900, 8 December 1975
S/12085, 26 May 1976

S/12093, 5 June 1976
S/12323, 30 April 1977
S/12723, 31 May 1978
S/13369, 31 May 1979
S/14100, 11 August 1980
S/14778, 1 December 1980
S/14490, 27 May 1981
S/15149, 1 June 1982
S/15502, 1 December 1982
S/15812, 1 June 1983
S/16148, 16 November 1983
S/16192, 1 December 1983
S/16519, 1 May 1984
S/16858, 12 December 1984
S/18102/Add. I, 11 June 1986
S/18491, 2 December 1986

General Assembly Resolutions

3212 (XXIX), 1 November 1974
3395 (XXX), 20 November 1975
3450, 9 December 1975
31/12, 12 November 1976
32/15, 9 November 1977
33/15, 9 November 1978
34/30, 20 November 1979
37/253, 13 May 1983

General Assembly Documents

A/8794, 27 September 1972
GA/4618-4622, 28 September 1972
A/32/133, 7 July 1977
A/33/113, 26 May 1978
A/33/233, 12 September 1978
A/38/586, 16 November 1983
A/41/96, 21 January 1986

U.N. Press Releases

SG/SM/1566-SC3259, 27 October 1971
SG/SM/1747, 12 September 1972
NV/318 (renumbered NV/319), 13 October 1972
NV/320, 20 October 1972
CYP/94/13

The United States

Controlling the Damage: US Policy Options for Greece. A Study Mission Report.

93rd Congress, 18-21 January 1974 (Washington, DC: US Government Printing Office, 1974).
Cyprus – 1974. Hearing. 93rd Congress, 2nd Session, 19-20 August 1974 (Washington, DC: US Government Printing Office, 1974).
Crisis on Cyprus: 1974. A Study Mission Report. 93rd Congress, 2nd Session, 14 October 1974 (Washington, DC: US Government Printing Office, 1974).
Crisis on Cyprus: 1975. One Year After the Invasion. 94th Congress, 2nd Session, 20 July 1975 (Washington, DC: US Government Printing Office, 1975).
Europe, South and East: Redefining the American Interest. Report. 94th Congress, 1st Session (Washington, DC: US Government Printing Office, 1975).
The Military Aspects of Banning Arms Aid to Turkey. Hearing. 95th Congress, 2nd Session, 28 June 1978 (Washington, DC: US Government Printing Office, 1978).
Turkey, Greece and NATO: The Strained Alliance. A Staff Report. 96th Congress, 2nd Session (Washington, DC: US Government Printing Office, 1980).
Perspectives on NATO's Southern Flank. Report. 96th Congress, 2nd Session (Washington, DC: US Government Printing Office, 1980).

The United Kingdom

Cyprus 1974: Hearings before the Committee on Foreign Affairs (London: HM Stationery Office, 1974).
The Select Committee on Cyprus: Minutes of Evidence. 19 February 1976, Session 1975-76 HC No. 206-i (London: HM Stationery Office, 1976).
Report of the Select Committee on Cyprus, together with the Proceedings of the Committee: Minutes of Evidence and Appendices. House of Commons, Session 1975-76, HC No. 331 (London: HM Stationery Office, 1976).
Report from the Select Committee on Cyprus: Observations by the Government. House of Commons, Session 1975-76, Cmnd. No. 6579 (London: HM Stationery Office, 1976).
Parliamentary Debates (House of Commons), 1964-86.
Parliamentary Debates (House of Lords), 1964-86.

Cyprus Government Press and Information Office

Cyprus Problem: The March 1986 'Draft Framework Agreement' and the Greek Cypriot side's attitude towards it (n.d.)
Turkish Demographic Manipulations in Cyprus (June 1987).
Cyprus Intercommunal Talks following the Turkish Invasion of July-August 1974 (October 1979).
The Cyprus Refugee Problem: Humanitarian Aspects (1989).
Cyprus, The True Percentage of the Turkish Cypriot Population (n.d.).
Turkish Expansionism (May 1987).
Turkish Colonization: A Threat for Cyprus and its People (n.d.).
Turkey and the Turkish Cypriots (n.d.).
Economic Integration of the Occupied Part of Cyprus with Turkey (July 1987).
Cyprus: A Question of Occupation, Colonization and Expansionism. An address

delivered by H.E. Mr George Iacovou, Minister of Foreign Affairs of the Republic of Cyprus before the South East Europe Society in Munich (n.d.).
Cyprus in Brief (1980).
The Refugees of Cyprus (n.d.).
The Oppression Myth and the Real Aim of Turkey in Cyprus (July 1987).
The Cyprus Problem (November 1989, revised).
Cyprus and the Non-Aligned Movement (April 1981, revised).
Turkish Policy on Cyprus and Efforts to Solve the Cyprus Problem (May 1989).
President Makarios's Last Public Speech and Press Conference (August 1987).
The American Arms Embargo Against Turkey, October 1979 (n.d.).
Certain Facts about the Cyprus Problem: An Analysis of Turkish Policy (June 1976).
Cyprus Intercommunal Talks. New Series, First Round. Vienna, 1 March-7 April 1977 (n.d.).
Documents handed by the Foreign Minister of the Republic of Cyprus to the UN Secretary-General in Geneva on 4 April 1979 (1979).
International Condemnation of the Turkish Cypriot Pseudostate (November 1989).

Cyprus Bar Association

Human Rights: Turkey's Violations of Human Rights in Cyprus (June 1989).

PANCYPRIAN COMMITTEE OF PARENTS AND RELATIVES OF UNDECLARED POW'S AND MISSING PERSONS

The Case of the Missing Cypriots (November 1987)
In Search of the Missing (undated)

Turkish-Cypriot Administration

Planning Bureau of the Provisional Cyprus Turkish Administration

United Nations Aid to Cyprus (March 1970).

'Turkish Federated State of Cyprus', Public Information Office

The Tragedy of Zyyi (April 1977).
Basic Facts about the Turkish Federated State of Cyprus (November 1979).

Historical Research Group, Cyprus

Chronology of Cyprus Conflict, 1878-1978 (September 1978).

Private Memoranda

Ertekun, Necati. 'A Memorandum on Efforts to Reach a Negotiated Settlement of the Cyprus Problem and the Constructive Role of the Turkish Cypriot Side to This End.'

Talk by Rauf Denktash to the Cyprus Sociological Association in March 1974.

INTERVIEWS

Some of the individuals interviewed do not wish to be named. The others are listed below.

Mr Rokoszewski, UNFICYP's Spokesman
Alper Ali-Riza, QC
George Vassiliou, the former President of Cyprus
Costa Carras, a founder member of the Committee of the 'Friends of Cyprus'
Sir Cyril Townsend
Dr Peter Loizos, Reader at the London School of Economics
Ozker Ozgur, former Leader of the Turkish Republican Party
Sotiris Georgalis, Press Counsellor, Cyprus High Commission, London
Glafkos Clerides, President of Cyprus
Michalakis Triantafyllides, former Attorney-General of Cyprus
Alper Gench, former Press Officer of the Office of 'TRNC' in London
Charles Goulkin, former spokesman of UNFICYP

NEWSPAPERS AND NEWS JOURNALS

Nea (Greece)
Cyprus Mail
Financial Times (London)
Avgi (Cyprus)
Alithia (Cyprus)
Simerini (Cyprus)
Agon (Cyprus)
The Times (London)
Hurriet (Turkey)
Sunday Times (London)
New York Times
Philelephtheros (Cyprus)
The Guardian (London)
The Economist (London)
Christian Science Monitor
Washington Post
Milliyet (Turkey)
Newsweek
Keesing's
The Middle East
Olay (Turkish Cypriot)

SECONDARY SOURCES

BOOKS AND DISSERTATIONS

Adams, T.W., and Alvin, J. Cottrell, *Cyprus between East and West* (Baltimore, MD: John Hopkins University Press, 1968).

Ahmed, Ferioz, *The Turkish Experiment in Democracy, 1960-1975* (London: Hurst, 1977).

Alasya, Halil Fikret, *The Republic of Cyprus and the events that have come to pass* (Ankara: Ayyildiz Matbaasi, 1969).

Attalides, Michael, *Cyprus: Nationalism and International Politics* (Edinburgh: Q Press, 1979).

Ball, George W., *The Past Has Another Pattern* (NewYork: W.W. Norton, 1982).

Birand, M.A., *30 Hot Days* (Istanbul: K. Rustem and Bro. 1985).

Bitsios, Dimitri S., *Cyprus: The Vulnerable Republic* (Thessaloniki: Institute for Balkan Studies, 1975).

Callaghan, James, *Time and Chance* (London: Collins, 1987).

Caradon, Lord, *Cyprus – Past and Future: A Personal Perspective* (Muncie, Indiana: Ball State University, 1980).

Clerides, Glafkos, *Cyprus: My Deposition*, 4 vols (Nicosia: Alithia, 1989-92).

Coufoudakis, Van (ed.), *Essays on the Cyprus Conflict* (New York: Pella, 1976).

Couloumbis, Theodore A., and Sallie M. Hicks, (eds), *U.S. Foreign Policy toward Greece and Cyprus: The Clash of Principle and Pragmatism* (Washington DC: Centre for Mediterranean Studies and American Hellenic Institute, 1975).

Crawshaw, Nancy, *The Cyprus Revolt: An Account of the Struggle for Union with Greece* (London: Geo. Allen and Unwin, 1978).

Critchley, Julian (ed.), *Cyprus: The Time Bomb of the Mediterranean*, (London: Atlantic Information Centre for Teachers, 1975).

Crossman, Richard, *The Diaries of a Cabinet Minister*, vol. II (London: Hamish Hamilton and Jonathan Cape, 1976).

Denktash, Rauf R., *The Cyprus Triangle* (Nicosia: K. Rustem and Bro., 2nd edn, 1988).

Ehrlich, Thomas, *International Crises and the Role of Law: Cyprus, 1958-1967* (Oxford University Press, 1974).

Ertekun, Necati Munir, *In Search of a Negotiated Cyprus Settlement* (Nicosia: ULUS Matbaachik, 1981).

——, *The Cyprus Dispute and the Birth of the Turkish Republic of Northern Cyprus* (Nicosia: K. Rustem and Bro., 2nd edn, 1984).

Evdokas, Takis, *The Symbiosis of the Two Communities* (Nicosia: Socio-Psychological Research Group, 1978).

Fallaci, Oriana, *Interview with History* (New York: Liveright, 1976, reprinted Boston: Houghton Mifflin, 1977).

Faulds, Andrew, *Excerpta Cypria For Today* (Nicosia: K. Rustem & Bro. 1988).

Feyzioglu, Turhan, and Necati M. Ertekun, *The Crux of the Cyprus question* (Nicosia: 1987).

Foley, Charles, and W.I. Scobie, *The Struggle for Cyprus* (Stanford, CA: Hoover Institution Press, 1975).

Foot, Michael, and Mervyn Jones, *Quietly Men 1957: Suez + Cyprus* (New York: Rinehart and Co., 1957).

Grivas, George, *The Memoirs of General Grivas* (transl. & ed. Charles Foley, London: Longman, 1964).

Harbottle, Michael, *The Impartial Soldier* (Oxford University Press, 1970).

Hare, A. Paul, *Cyprus – Conflict and Resolution* (University of Cape Town, 1974).

Hitchens, Christopher, *Cyprus* (London: Quartet, 1984).

Ikle, F.C., *How Nations Negotiate* (New York: Harper and Row, 1964).

Jacovides, Andreas J., *The Cyprus Question: Its Dimensions, Implications and Prospects for a Solution* (Washington, DC: Centre for Mediterranean Studies, 1980).

——, *A View from Within: the Role of Small States and the Cyprus Experiences* (Nicosia: Public Information Office, 1969).

James, Alan, *Peacekeeping in International Politics* (London: Macmillan, 1990).

Joseph, Suad, and Barbara L.K. Pillsbury (eds), *Muslim-Christian Conflicts: Economic, Political and Social Origins* (Boulder, CO: Westview Press, 1978).

Kaloudis, George, S., 'The Role of the UN in Cyprus from 1964 to 1979' (unpubl. Ph.D. thesis, University of Kansas, 1982).

Karpat, Kemal H., *Turkey's Foreign Policy in Transition, 1950-1974* (Leiden: E.J. Brill, 1975).

Kedourie, Elie, *The Cyprus Problem and its Solution* (Rome: Centre for Mediterranean Studies, American Universities Field Staff, 1974).

Kosut, Hal, *Cyprus, 1946-68* (New York: Facts on File, 1970).

Kuchuk, Fazil, *The Cyprus Question, A Permanent Solution* (Nicosia, 1957).

Kyprianou, Spyros, *The Cyprus Question: The British Reply to the British* (Athens: National Committee for Self-Determination of Cyprus, 1956).

Kyriakides, Stanley, *Cyprus Constitutionalism and Crisis Government* (Philadelphia: University of Pennsylvania Press, 1968).

Kyrris, Costas P., *Peaceful Co-existence in Cyprus under British Rule (1878-1959) and after Independence: An Outline* (Nicosia, 1977).

——, *History of Cyprus* (Nicosia: Nicocles, 1985).

Lantitis, N.C., *Our Destiny* (Nicosia: the author, 1963).

Levine, Edward Philip, 'The Mediation of International Disputes' (unpubl. Ph.D. thesis, Yale University, 1971).

Lewis, G., *Modern Turkey* (London: Ernest Benn, 1974).

Mackenzie, Kenneth, *Cyprus: The Ideological Crucible* (London: Institute for the Study of Conflict, 1972).

Markides, Kyriascos C., *The Rise and Fall of the Cyprus Republic* (New Haven: Yale University Press, 1977).

Mayes, Stanley, *Makarios: A Biography* (London: Macmillan, 1981).

Mouzelis, N.P., *Modern Greece: Facets of Underdevelopment* (London: Macmillan, 1978).

Necatigil, Zaim M., *The Cyprus Question and the Turkish Position in International Law* (Oxford University Press, 1989).

Nicolson, Harold, *Diaries and Letters, 1945-62* (esp. letter to Juliet Nicolson, 31 July 1954) (London: Collins, 1968).

Oberling, Pierre, *The Road to Bellapaise: The Turkish Cypriot Exodus to Northern*

Cyprus (Social Science Monographs, Boulder, CO, distributed by Columbia University Press, 1982).

Panteli, Stavros, *The Making of Modern Cyprus: From Obscurity to Statehood* (New Barnet: Interworld, 1990).

Papandreou, Andreas, *Democracy at Gunpoint* (Garden City: Doubleday, 1970).

Patrick, Richard A., *Political Geography and the Cyprus Conflict: 1963-1971* (University of Waterloo, Ontario, Department of Geography, publication series 4, 1976).

Polyviou, Polyvios G., *Cyprus in Search of a Constitution* (Nicosia: Nicolaou, 1976), esp. Part II, Chapter IV.

——, *Cyprus: Conflict and Negotiation, 1960-1980* (London: Duckworth, 1980).

Reddaway, John, *Burdened with Cyprus: The British Connection* (London: Weidenfeld & Nicolson, 1986).

Royal Institute of International Affairs, Information Department, *Cyprus: The Dispute and the Settlement* (London: RIIA, Chatham House Memoranda, 1964).

Rusinow, Dennison I., *The Cyprus Deadlock: Forever or Another Day*? (Hanover, NH: American Universities Field Staff, 1981).

Ryan, Stephen, 'Ethnic Conflict and the International System: Foreign Involvement in the Cyprus Problem, 1974-1982' (unpubl. Ph.D. thesis, London School of Economics, 1984).

Salih, Halil Ibrahim, *Cyprus: An Analysis of the Cypriot Political Discord* (Brooklyn, NY: Theo Gaus, 1968).

—, *Cyprus: The Impact of Diverse Nationalism on a State* (University of Alabama Press, 1978).

Soylemez, Yuksel, *Foreign Policy of Turkey at the United Nations* (Ankara: Ministry of Foreign Affairs, vol. 1, 1973).

Stavrinides, Zenon, *The Cyprus Conflict: National Identity and Statehood* (Nicosia: Loris Stavrinides), 1976.

Stearns, Monteagle, *Entangled Allies: US Policy towards Greece, Turkey and Cyprus* (New York: Council on Foreign Relations Press, 1992).

Stegenga, James A., *The United Nations Force in Cyprus* (Columbus: Ohio State University Press for the Mershon Centre for Education in National Security, 1968).

Stephens, Robert, *Cyprus: A Place of Arms* (London: Pall Mall Press, 1966).

Stern, L., *The Wrong Horse: The Politics of Intervention and the Failure of American Diplomacy* (New York: Times Books, 1978).

Stevens, Carl M., *Strategy and Collective Bargaining Negotiations* (New York: McGraw-Hill, 1963).

Stoessinger, John G., *The United Nations and the Superpowers: China, Russia and America* (New York: Random House, 3rd edn, 1973).

Tamkoc, Metin, *The Turkish Cypriot State: The Embodiment of the Right of Self-determination* (Nicosia: K. Rustem & Bro., 1988).

Tremayne, Penelope, *Below the Tide* (London: Hutchinson, 1958).

Tuncliff, K.H., 'The United Nations and the Mediation of International Conflict' (unpubl. Ph.D. thesis, University of Iowa, 1984).

Vanezis, P.N., *Makarios: Faith and Power* (London: Abelard-Schuman, 1971).

—, *Makarios: Pragmatism versus Idealism* (London: Ableard-Schuman, 1974).

——, *Makarios: Life and Leadership* (London: Abelard-Schuman, 1971).

Volkan, Vamik D., *Cyprus – War and Adaptation: A Psychoanalytic History of Two Ethnic Groups in Conflict* (Charlottesville: University of Virginia Press, 1979).

Waldheim, Kurt, *The Challenge of Peace* (London: Weidenfeld and Nicolson, 1980).

Weiner, Sharon Anderholm, 'Turkish Foreign Policy Decision Making on the Cyprus Issue: A Comparative Analysis of Three Crises' (unpubl. Ph.D. thesis, Duke University, 1980).

Weintal, E., and A. Bartlett, *Facing the Brink: An Intimate Study of Crisis Diplomacy* (New York, Charles Scribner's Sons, 1967).

Windsor, Philip, *NATO and the Cyprus Crisis* (London: Institute for Strategic Studies, Adelphi Papers, 14, 1964).

Wittner, L., *American Intervention in Greece* (New York: Columbia University Press, 1982).

Worsley, Peter, and Paschalis Kitromilides (eds), *Small States in the Modern World: The Conditions of Survival* (Nicosia: Cyprus Sociological Association and New Cyprus Association, 1979).

Xydis, Stephen G., *Cyprus Conflict and Conciliation, 1954-1958* (Columbus: Ohio State University Press for the Mershon Centre for Education in National Security, 1967).

——, *Cyprus: Reluctant Republic* (The Hague, Paris: Mouton, 1973).

ARTICLES AND CHAPTERS IN BOOKS

Acheson, Dean, 'Cyprus: the Anatomy of the Problem', *Chicago Bar Record* (46, 8, May 1965), pp. 349-56.

Adams, T.W., 'The American Concern in Cyprus', *Annals of the American Academy of Political and Social Science* (401, May 1972), pp. 95-105.

Adams, T.W., and Alvin J. Cottrell, 'American Foreign Policy and the UN Peacekeeping Force in Cyprus', *Orbis* (12, 2, summer 1968), pp. 490-503.

——, 'Communism in Cyprus', *Problems of Communism* (vol. 15, 3, May-June 1966), pp. 22-30.

Attalides, Michael, 'The Turkish Cypriots: Their Relations to the Greek Cypriots in Perspective' in Michael Attalides (ed.), *Cyprus Reviewed* (Nicosia: Jus Cypri Association, 1977).

Australian Foreign Affairs Record, 'The Cyprus Dispute and the Search for a Settlement' (October 1977), pp. 496-501.

Aziz, Dundar, 'The Cyprus Situation', *Pakistan Horizon* (XXVIII, 2, 1975), p. 16.

Barkun, B., 'Conflict Resolution Through Implicit Mediation', *Journal of Conflict Resolution* (8, 1964), pp. 121-30.

Barston, R.P., 'The Foreign Policy of Cyprus' in R.P. Barston (ed.), *The Other Powers: Studies in Foreign Policies of Small States* (London: Geo. Allen & Unwin; New York: Harper and Row, 1973).

Bowyer Bell, J., 'Violence at a Distance: Greece and the Cyprus Crisis', *Orbis* (18, 3, fall 1974), pp. 791-808.

Boyd, James M., 'Cyprus: Episode in Peacekeeping', *International Organization* (vol. 20, no. 1, 1966), pp. 1-17.

Bruce, Leigh H., 'Cyprus. A Last Chance', *Foreign Policy* (58, spring 1985), pp. 115-33.

Camp, Glen D., 'Greek-Turkish Conflict Over Cyprus', *Political Science Quarterly* (95, 1, spring 1980), pp. 43-70.

——, ms. prepared for *Polity, Journal of the Northeast Political Science Association* (1988).

——, 'Cyprus Between the Powers: 1980-1989', *Cyprus Review* (Nicosia: Intercollege, 1, 2, fall 1989), pp. 65-90.

Coufoudakis, Van, 'Defining Greek Foreign Policy Objectives' in Howard R. Penniman (ed.), *Greece at the Polls: The National Elections of 1974 and 1977* (Washington, DC: American Enterprise Institute for Public Policy Research, 1981).

——, 'Greek Political Party Attitudes Towards Turkey: 1974-89' in Dimitri Constas (ed.), *The Greek-Turkish Conflict in the 1990s* (London, Macmillan, 1991).

——, 'United Nations Peacekeeping and Peacemaking and the Cyprus Question', *Western Political Quarterly* (29[3], 9, 1976), pp. 457-73.

——, 'United States Foreign Policy and the Cyprus Question: A Case Study in Cold War Diplomacy' in Michael Attalides (ed.), *Cyprus Reviewed* (Nicosia: Jus Cypri Association, 1977).

——, 'U.S. Foreign Policy and the Cyprus Question: An Interpretation', *Millenium: Journal of International Studies* (5, 3, winter 1976-7), pp. 245-68.

Crawshaw, Nancy, 'Cyprus: A Failure in Western Diplomacy', *The World Today* (40, 2, February 1984), pp. 73-8.

——, 'Cyprus after Makarios: Prospects for a Settlement', *The World Today* (34, 1, January 1978), pp. 31-8.

Current Digest of the Soviet Press (38, 3, 19 February 1986), pp. 16-17.

Cutler, Robert, 'Soviet Relations with Greece and Turkey: A Systems Perspective' in Dimitri Constas (ed.), *The Greek- Turkish Conflict in the 1990s* (London: Macmillan, 1991).

Denktash, Rauf R., 'The Problem of Cyprus', *Review of International Affairs* (Yugoslavia, 22, 544, 5 December 1972), pp. 9-11.

Dobell, W.M., 'Division over Cyprus', *International Journal* (22, 2, spring 1967), pp. 278-92.

Drooz, Daniel B., 'Cyprus: The 'Quiet' Civil War', *Times of Israel* (1, 5, April 1974), pp. 42-7.

Evriviades, Marios L., 'The Problem of Cyprus', *Current History* (70, 412, January 1976), pp. 18-21 and 38-42).

Fisher, Roger, 'Fractioning Conflict' in Roger Fisher (ed.), *International Conflict and Behavioural Sciences: The Craigville Papers* (New York: Basic Books, 1964).

Haas, Richard N., 'Cyprus Moving beyond Solution', *Washington Quarterly* (10, 2, spring 1987), pp. 183-90.

Hale, William, 'Turkey's Inconclusive Election', *The World Today* (33, 7, July 1977) pp. 243-7.

Harding, Lord of Petherton, 'The Cyprus Problem in Relation to the Middle East', *International Affairs* (34, 3, July 1958), pp. 291-6.

Hitchens, Christopher, 'Detente and Destabilization: Report from Cyprus', *New Left Review* (94, November-December 1975), pp. 61-73.

Hughes, James, 'The Cypriot Labyrinth', *New Left Review* (29, January-February 1965), pp. 41-52.

Ikle, Fred Charles and Nathan Leites, 'Political Negotiation as a Process of Modifying Utilities', *Journal of Conflict Resolution* (6, 1, March 1962), pp. 19-28.

Jacovides, Andreas J., 'The Cyprus Problem and the United Nations' in Michael Attalides (ed.), *Cyprus Reviewed* (Nicosia: Jus Cypri Association, 1977).

Joseph, Joseph S., 'The UN as an Instrument of National Policy: The Case of Cyprus', *Cyprus Review* (Nicosia: Intercollege, 1, 2, fall 1989), pp. 46-65.

Keashly, Loraleigh, 'Towards a Contingency Approach to Third Party Intervention in Regional Conflict: A Cyprus Illustration', *International Journal* (XLV, spring 1990), pp. 424-53.

Kemp, Peter, 'Cyprus', *Middle East Economic Digest* (34/37, 21 September 1990), pp. 9-15.

——, (35/35, 6 September 1992), pp. 13-18.

Laipson, Helen, 'US Policy Towards Greece and Turkey Since 1974' in Dimitri Constas (ed.), *The Greek-Turkish Conflict in the 1990s* (London: Macmillan, 1991).

Loizos, Peter, 'The Progress of Greek Nationalism in Cyprus, 1878-1970' in J. Davis (ed.), *Choice and Change: Essays in Honour of Lucy Mair* (London School of Economics, 1974).

Lumsden, Malvern, 'The Cyprus Conflict as a Prisoner's Dilemma Game', *Journal of Conflict Resolution* (17, 1, March 1973), pp. 7-32.

Mandic, Nicola, 'Cyprus After Makarios', *Review of International Affairs* (XXVIII, 660, 5 October 1977), p. 26.

Mayes, Stanley, 'Can the Cyprus Problem be Solved?', *The Round Table* (273, January 1979), pp. 81-7.

McDonald, Robert, 'Cyprus: The UN Tries Again', *The World Today* (40, 10, October 1984), p. 420.

——, 'Cyprus: The Gulf Widens', *The World Today* (42, 11, November 1986), p. 185.

Michaelides, Alecos, 'The House of Representatives of the Republic of Cyprus', *Parliamentarian* (60, 2, April 1979), pp. 67-71.

Miller, W., 'A New Era in Greece', *Foreign Affairs* (14, 4, July 1936), pp. 654-61.

Navarro, Christina K., 'Cyprus and the U.N.: A Case for Non- military Collective Measures', *Indiana Law Journal* (54, 1, 1978-9), pp. 125-63.

Pipinelis, Panayotis, 'The Greco-Turkish Feud Revived', *Foreign Affairs* (37, 2, January 1959), pp. 306-16.

Pollis, Adamandia, 'Intergroup Conflict and British Colonial Policy: The Case of Cyprus', *Comparative Politics* (5, 4, July 1973), pp. 575-99.

Psomiades, Harry J., 'The Cyprus Dispute', *Current History* (43, 285, May 1965), pp. 269-76 and 305-6.

Rikhye, Indar Jit, 'Peace-making, Non-Violence and Truth', *International Peace Academy Reports* (33, June 1973), p. 8.

Rosenbaum, Naomi, 'Cyprus and the United Nations: An Appreciation of Parliamentary Diplomacy', *Canadian Journal of Economics and Political Science* (33, 1967), pp. 218-31.

——, 'Success in Foreign Policy: The British in Cyprus, 1878-1960', *Canadian Journal of Political Science* (3, 4, December 1970), pp. 605-27.

Round Table, The, 'Enosis and its Background: Race and Religion in Cyprus' (42, 186, March 1957), pp. 129-40.

Rudnick, David, 'NATO and the Cyprus Crisis', *The Round Table* (266, April 1977), pp. 182-90.

Shepard, H.A., 'Responses to Situations of Competition and Conflict' in Elise Boulding (ed.), *Conflict Management in Organizations* (Ann Arbor: University of Michigan Press, 1961).

Snyder, Jed C., 'Strategic Bias and Southern Flank Security', *Washington Quarterly* (8, 3, summer 1985) pp. 123-36.

Souter, David, 'An Island Apart: A Review of the Cyprus Problem', *Third World Quarterly* (6, 3, July 1984), pp. 657-74.

Stegenga, James A., 'UN Peacekeeping: The Cyprus Venture', *Journal of Peace Research* (7, 1970), pp. 1-15.

Stern, Laurence, 'Bitter Lessons: How we failed in Cyprus', *Foreign Policy* (19, summer 1975), pp. 34-78.

Thomas, Ann van Wynen, and A.J. Thomas, 'The Cyprus Crisis 1974-75: Political and Juridical Aspects', *Southwestern Law Journal* (29, 1975), pp. 513-46.

Varrier, Anthony, 'Cyprus: Britain's Security Role', *The World Today* (20, 3, March 1964), pp. 131-7.

Xydis, Stephen G., 'Toward "Toil and Moil" in Cyprus', *Middle East Journal* (20, 1, winter 1966), pp. 1-19.

Yegorov, B., 'Just and Lasting Settlement for Cyprus', *International Affairs* (Moscow, 11, November 1984), pp. 71-9.

INDEX